FACING MY GIANTS

Overcoming Obstacles for Optimal Health

Dawn G. Green

FACING MY GIANTS: OVERCOMING OBSTACLES FOR
OPTIMAL HEALTH
BY DAWN G. GREEN

Published by Green Living
ISBN:979-8-9886573-0-9
Library of Congress Control Number: 2023914457

Cover design by Elite Authors
Interior design by Never Alone Publishing

Available in print and as an e-book from amazon.com.
For more information on this book and the author, visit
www.greenlivinginc.com.

Printed in the United States of America.

This book is dedicated to all my readers
who are suffering from chronic diseases,
whose voices have gone unheard.
May the words inscribed within these pages
resonate loudly and clearly,
affecting a transformative change for us all.

CONTENTS

FOREWORD

RISING ABOVE ADVERSITY

Life is full of surprises, some of which we could never predict. Amidst the ups and downs, we can find ourselves at a loss for how to proceed when faced with adversity. For many of us, these hardships cause us to feel weak, vulnerable, and isolated. However, in these moments we become aware of the incredible strength embedded in us.

As you read this book, each chapter will provide intimate insights into overcoming adversity. No two challenges are alike. But the strength and resilience demonstrated in each person's story shows us that no matter what the obstacle, we can all find the *strength* to move forward.

Dawn Green's bravery cannot be overstated. She has faced multiple and extreme challenges in her life and has shown us that adversity, no matter how difficult, can be tackled and learned from. There is always a way forward.

Adversity can come from many sources and in many stages throughout our lives, both physical and emotional. It can be difficult to navigate these experiences alone, and often these circumstances require assistance and support from others. As you read through the chapters of this book, I encourage you to not only be inspired but also to seek out a community to support your challenges. Developing this community support system may be a different process for everyone, but it is an important step in overcoming adversity.

Whether struggling with disease, addiction, poverty, physical impairments, or simply the challenges of everyday life, one thing is certain: in the face of adversity, we find out who we *truly* are. We discover strengths we didn't know we possessed and develop a newfound appreciation for the world around us. This book encourages us to reflect upon our own experiences and hardships, to draw strength from them, and to recognize that we are all capable of taking control of our lives.

The author of this incredible book has not only proven her resilience by overcoming adversity in her life but has generously shared her story with you with the intention that it might inspire others searching for help and guidance while facing their own adversity.

As we discover these incredible stories of resilience and fortitude, let us take a moment to reflect on our own capacity for resilience. Let this book encourage us to remember that in difficult times, we all have an internal strength that can be found if we dig deep enough. We must never give up and never forget that we all have the ability to rise up, to heal, and to grow, no matter what difficulties we encounter.

It is my belief that no matter who you are or what challenges you are facing, everyone can find something to relate to within these pages. Each chapter provides insight into extraordinary perseverance and courage in the face of incredible difficulties.

Let us celebrate the remarkable author, Dawn Green, who has shared her journey with us and who offers an intimate glimpse into her life. Her story exemplifies how humans have the strength through God to adapt, to grow, and to overcome even the most challenging obstacles.

I invite you to join me as we embark on a journey of resilience and strength, where we'll find the courage to overcome adversity. Let the experiences in each chapter remind you of the powerful potential that we all possess to manifest positive change in our lives and the lives of those around us. Let us take each challenge to heart and *embrace* the realities of our experiences with authenticity, empathy, and unwavering strength.

Diana Martin-Gotcher, PhD
Holistic Life Coach, Author of *Raw Diligence*

PREFACE

In this world, there are all types of giants—tech giants, corporate giants, religious giants, and political giants. In my world, there are also sick giants. After thirty-five years of being misdiagnosed, my primary care physician (PCP) finally listened to me and ordered a specific test that provided an answer to the myriad of symptoms that had plagued me for decades. The unending appointments filled with frustration and unsympathetic responses finally resulted in hope, after my concerns were finally acknowledged and acted upon. That pivotal moment when the long-awaited test results came in led to a turning point in my healing journey. I finally had a name for what had been plaguing me all these years.

My continuous pain, both physically and emotionally, became my purpose, leading me on a journey of exploration and a personal plan of wellness that I specifically tailored to meet my unique needs.

I wrote this book because I wanted my journey to be a beacon of hope and light to you—those who are dealing with unexplained illnesses or those who know of a loved one or friend who is constantly sick and looking for additional modalities for discovering health. Each time I share my story in public or private, I am given the same mandate: "you must tell your story so that you can help others."

I so desperately wanted to wait until my story was picture perfect before I unleashed the raw details of my experience to you, but family and friends refused to allow me to delay it by continuously encouraging me to share my story with you now. I am most grateful to them for that.

This book was birthed out of my daily journal entries. I kept copious records of everything I experienced from the time I received my diagnoses until the writing of this book. When I started seeing the slightest signs of my body responding in ways that it never had in the six decades I had been alive, I knew then that I must stay the course on this treacherous terrain to do what I had never done to get the results that I had never received. I do not share my story with the intent that you would emulate what I have done. I share my story with the hope that you will find the courage to explore your unique body to learn what works best for you, then navigate through the tools I have shared so you too can take charge of your well-being and overcome your obstacles for optimal health.

Dawn G. Green
Librarian, Teacher, Researcher

ACKNOWLEDGMENTS

To *Yeshua*, the Great Physician, who kept me alive through all of the misdiagnoses.

To my mom, Annie, I wish you were here to see the answer to your relentless prayer.

To my husband, Lewis, you have been my caretaker from day one. Your selfless love is unmatched. There's a crown waiting for you in Glory.

To my daughter, Mikayla, it is my highest honor to be your mother. I love you to eternity and back. Taking care of you has consistently delayed the writing of this book.

To Dion and Belinda, there are no words to describe who you are to me. You have given of yourself more times than I can even count.

To Charlene, it is because of you that my story is even in print. You have urged me for years to tell my story to the world. Your love and support are the reasons this is a reality.

To Beverly, thank you for your constant love and understanding. I will never forget when you called me from Israel when I was going through my darkest hour of despair. "Me and you, us never part."[1]

To Sandy, you have consistently told me what you see in me. Your encouragement has propelled me to "fight the good fight of faith" (1 Timothy 6:12 NKJV).

To Val, thank you for always texting to check in on me even when I was too sick to text back.

To Pam, your love for me is palpable. I'm so happy to call you my sister.

To Mike and Lynn, I will always love you.

Chapter One

The Journey Begins

Healing takes courage, and we all have courage, even if we have to dig a little to find it.[2]

~Tori Amos

The journey of healing began to unfold when I went for what seemed like a routine mammogram. Since the age of twenty-seven, each year, when the earth completely orbits the sun, I have scheduled my exam. Unbeknownst to me, this one isolated event amidst all the other events of my life would change the trajectory of my essence. Everything I have prayed for and worked for concerning healing, health, and wholeness was about to meet destiny in a new and extraordinary way. What seemed customary to me was wrapped up in a divine appointment.

On the surface, the entire process appeared to be a setback, but by taking a closer look, I can see the Creator's handiwork plotting and charting a plan that to the undiscerning eye looked like pure defeat. I've heard many sermons where the pastor said, "Your greatest gift is sometimes wrapped up in your biggest problem." Looking at the circumstances of my life and how trials and hard times have played out, hearing that sentiment repeatedly has resonated so strongly with me.

By nature, I am an optimistic person, and that statement holds much weight when I view my life through the lens of all I've gone through. If you were in my inner circle, you would have seen how I relentlessly fought giant after giant. Some seemed like they would overtake me, but amazingly, in the end, I miraculously overcame them.

Every routine breast exam appeared to get the best of me. I was often filled with trepidation right before the mammogram because in my breasts, as far back as I can remember, I have

1

experienced excruciating pain, and each visit seemed to aggravate it—especially in my left breast.

When I first entered puberty and started to develop breasts, I often told my mom that my breasts hurt. Each time she lovingly said, "They are hurting because you are growing." Somehow, she equated the pain with growing pains. The many years they hurt made it seem as if the pain was a part of me. Essentially, it had become a part of my life. There was never a day my breasts did not hurt. Some days were worse than others. As I got older, I asked close friends probing questions to find out if they too had experienced painful breasts, and they all concurred that if they did have pain, it was only around the time of their menstruation.

Despite the pain, I faithfully made my appointment at the doctor's office for this very important screening. Even if the pain was severe, I still courageously went. This day proved to be no different. I mustered up the strength and courage to brave the pain, then return home to wait patiently for the results.

A Horrific Phone Call

A few days following the mammogram, I received a horrific phone call. During the call, the doctor informed me that another lump was discovered in that same painful left breast. When my home phone rang and the speaker on the caller ID announced the person on the line, my heart raced uncontrollably. *Oh boy, here we go.* I did not want to pick up the phone for fear of the news I might receive.

Instead of answering the phone right away, I paced back and forth in my kitchen, staring at the phone as if the person on the other end could see me being frantic, and I prayed that they would break the news to me gently. All the while, I wished my husband, Lew, was home with me to soften the blow of what I thought I was about to hear. Incomprehensible fear kept me from answering the phone. However, after the phone's third announcement, I snapped out of my stupor and rushed to grab the phone, almost knocking over my countertop bar stools.

Although I had hesitated at first, my current goal was to pick up the receiver before the allotted rings on the phone ended and the message went to voicemail. I most certainly did not want the person on the other end to leave me a grim message time-stamped on my answering machine forever. I also feared that if I did not pick up the phone right away, I would have to give the hospital a call back, which might result in getting their voicemail message and delaying the news of my results even further.

The bottom line is that I knew I had to pick up the phone and face my fears head on. In that short span of debating whether I should answer the phone, I was simultaneously bracing myself for what I was about to hear on the other end of that phone. The scenario created an unbelievable level of stress.

A call from the doctor or hospital after any routine test is usually a reliable indication that it is not going to be good news. No doctor has ever called me to say, "Guess what? Everything is just fine." In my experience, any good news is delivered in a letter, but the bad news oftentimes warrants a phone call.

When I finally answered the phone, the caller said, "Please state your name and date of birth." The salutation alone let me know this was serious official medical business. After I coherently gave that factual identifiable information, the caller informed me of the call's purpose. The shaking in my voice and slurred words unequivocally signaled her that I was quite nervous. I wanted to scream and blurt out, "Excuse me, miss. I'm scared."

Somehow the caller was moved with compassion as she shared the diagnosis, and she mercifully assured me they would take good care of me. She told me what the mammogram had revealed and that the hospital had a new machine, which could take a 360° diagnostic mammogram and give them even more accurate and detailed information about the nature of the lump. This machine, she said, could provide ironclad confirmation of their findings.

As we continued to speak, my fear of another painful mammogram set in. The excruciating pain in my breast had intensified. Years of getting to know my own body and being more aware of its nuances have taught me that I carry most of my stress

3

in my left breast. Anytime I hear bad news, I feel the brunt of it in my breast.

As the phone conversation continued, fear fully took over. I was repulsed by the fact I was required to get another mammogram. All I could feel was unbearable pain emanating from my breast and coursing through my entire body.

At that moment, everything went black. My thinking became impaired, and I could no longer speak coherently. I could not bear to have another painful mammogram. As she was talking, I wondered, *Why won't they just give me an ultrasound since the lump has already been found? Why go back and look again? What are they looking for?*

I continued to listen to her explain further what this new machine could see and detect. Every time I said, "But we already have the results of a mammogram. Why do we need another one?," she rebutted with "This is procedure." Reluctantly, I agreed to have a second mammogram, mainly because I felt I had no other choice. I wanted and needed answers to what was going on with my health, so I decided to face the inevitable and not to delay it by trying to persuade her this second mammogram seemed unnecessary.

The nurse asked me to stay on the line while she checked the availability of a time slot. Usually, mammograms are scheduled weeks in advance. Fortunately, a spot was available in the upcoming week. She put me on the official schedule for this state-of-the-art mammography.

A Comforting Call

When my call with the nurse ended, I dialed Lew's cell phone. The moment he answered, a bottled-up suppressed cry emanated from my soul that shook him to his core. Once I released all that tension, I whispered the words, "The hospital just called."

There was dead silence on the other end, then he quietly said, "And what did they say?"

"Another lump was found."

Lew guaranteed me that together we would get through this like we had gotten through so many other things. I believed him because we have a track record together. He has been in this fight

4

with me for all of our marriage. At the time of this writing, that is thirty-two years.

It has always been us against the world. He is the epitome of loving your wife "as Christ loved the church" (Ephesians 5:25 NIV). He has laid down his life to ensure my well-being comes first. I often share with him that I am not able to repay him for sacrificially loving me, but a reward from our heavenly Father awaits him for going the distance with me from day one. It's one thing to take care of your spouse who gets sick after you get married, but it's a whole different level of love when you marry someone knowing full well your partner is chronically ill. That day, his faith-filled assuring words comforted me as they had on many other occasions. But as I've often experienced, peace was temporary. Fear set in with a vengeance.

"Here Comes Another One"

The day of the scheduled 360° mammogram finally arrived. At the hospital, the receptionist checked me in and escorted me to a tiny room, filled with approximately ten grimacing women who appeared to be at least twenty to thirty years older than I was. When I saw their faces, my heart sank. Everything about what I saw and felt seemed so unfair. Everyone appeared to be at the mercy of someone else, as if their happiness and fate were linked directly to a test result.

When I walked through the doorway, some looked up and some did not, but their expressions said, "Here comes another one." I longed for the private room I had grown accustomed to at the hospital I frequented when I lived in New Jersey. The uneasiness of being called back for a second mammogram made me want to be in a room by myself so I would not have to look at those somber faces.

As an empath, I intuitively pick up the energy in a room. I feel what others are feeling, and most recently, I have been trying to soften the blows of other people's emotions by being more aware of how this affects me and by using my knowledge to deflect negative energy so I do not take it upon myself. This is yet another tool in my tool chest I have learned to use for my advantage and for my total well-being on this healing journey.

In the room that day, I could not bear to see such despair on the other women's faces as they awaited their test results. My heart was already melancholy, yet I was laboring to be optimistic inwardly and outwardly. Due to the room's size, the chairs were positioned in a way that once you took your seat, you were forced to look into the eyes of each woman unless you elected to keep your head down the whole time you waited for your name to be called. The place was like a hotel with a revolving door: as one was called to hear her results, another was brought in. The whole scene was reminiscent of a dystopian novel I had read during my tenure as a middle school librarian. The fear was palpable.

All the women housed in that cramped space hoped to hear a positive word concerning their screening. As I walked past the women on my way to a tiny cubicle to change, I was given a directive by the nurse who escorted me. She specifically said to undress from the waist up and put on a gown with the opening in the front. She also instructed me to place my belongings in a drawstring plastic bag, provided compliments of the hospital, and bring the bag with me when my name was called. I did exactly as I was told. When I completed her verbal checklist, I tightly clutched my drawstring bag and took my seat in the circle to join my fellow comrades, while I waited for the nurse to return and rescue me from this awful place.

The atmosphere was thick. The overwhelming somberness made it feel as if there was literally no oxygen left in the room. To lighten the heaviness, I started a conversation with a group of ladies sitting closest to me. I do not recall what I said, but I made them laugh. It felt good to break the ice. I claimed a kind of victory, knowing I would not leave the room the way I found it. If no one else felt better, I sure did. As I mentally geared up for the state-of-the-art diagnostic mammogram, I wanted to avoid the buildup of pain in my left breast that tension caused. Laughter always helped.

While the other women and I enjoyed our laughter, the door opened. The nurse stood in the doorway with clipboard in hand and called out, "Green, Dawn Green, come with me." I gladly maneuvered my way out of that small room to follow the nurse down the hall to the examination room. I was thankful for the good chuckle I shared with the ladies who were waiting for their name to be called, but the levity was not nearly enough to remove the intense pain. The pain was so jarring I felt its effects all the way to my backbone.

Cruel and Unusual Punishment

In the mammography room, I told the technician I was experiencing unbearable discomfort. I quickly tried to educate her about my situation and informed her I had several cysts, which may have contributed to the unusual pain. She didn't seem to be concerned with my medical history; she just stared at me blank-faced. I was trying desperately to evoke some level of compassion in her so that when my breast was squeezed between the plexiglass, she might not put too much pressure on the paddle compressor because I was already hurting beyond belief. But no response or concern emanated from her whatsoever.

I am always the most frightened when my life is placed in the hands of those who do not seem to care or have compassion. In between each breast image, I tried to convince the technician that my engorged breast being smashed as flat as a pancake between the plexiglass was causing unthinkable pain that made me want to drop to my knees. Her only response was "Hold your breath until I say 'breathe' and stay still."

I grunted and groaned in pain several times during the screening, but she ignored me. She had a job to do, but I felt this unusual circumstance needed a different approach. At one point, tears ran down my cheeks, yet I could not wipe them away because I had to "hold my breath and stay still." If I moved for even a millisecond, the image could be affected, and she would have to take another image. For me that was not a viable option. I had to stand there, take the pain, and get it over with. I could not survive a redo. I had no other recourse, because I did not want to have her repeat that painful process.

When the mammogram was completed, I was compelled to speak up. I said, "I am not a person who ever complains, but I am in horrific pain, and each time you placed the sharp edge of the plexiglass right on the lump you were trying to get a picture of and brought the machine down on my breast, I didn't know if I could even bear the pain, thus the tears streaming down my face."

Without uttering one word, she motioned me to the exit door and brought me back to the tiny room again. This time I was given the directive to not put my clothes back on until the radiologist confirmed no other pictures were needed. Maybe you can imagine my dismay. All I could think of is that no one cared about my pain or my feelings. The technician only wanted to complete a task. Anything else was off script and to be ignored. The technician's reaction to what I had just shared seemed so cold and aloof. Under my breath, I said, "Wow! This is cruel and unusual punishment no one deserves. No woman should ever have to suffer through this."

Another Mammogram?

Throughout my journey toward optimal health, I have wished there was a different kind of screening for people like me who suffer with sore, tender breasts. After waiting in that cramped room for what seemed like an eternity, I was escorted to an even smaller office to hear the report of what the new machine had found. The mass was indeed a cyst, and the surgeon wanted to aspirate it right away.

I was relieved to know I was going to be fine. Breast aspirations had become a normal routine. In my twenties, I had my first breast aspiration, so I knew what to expect. Before leaving the hospital, I was brought to another room to meet with the scheduler, who gave me my appointment and instructions for what to do before and after a cyst aspiration.

The day arrived for the cyst to be removed. I had to be at the hospital at 7:00 a.m. Excited for this early appointment, I calculated the approximate time I would be back home. I took joy in the fact that the outpatient procedure should not take long, and I could return home by 10:00 a.m. to rest and recover both mentally and physically. Getting back home and putting my feet up was a very welcoming idea. Maybe I could finally exhale.

When Lew and I arrived, we were the only ones in the waiting room. That was a good sign. The first one in and the first one out. But by 8:00 a.m., I still had not been called. The clerk at the front desk told us she would call us shortly. As each hour passed, Lew and I became more nervous. He had to go to work, and I wanted to get home to recover from my traumatic experience. The nervous energy bounced back and forth between us. His myriad of questions regarding why I was told to be there at 7:00 a.m. but was not called back yet made my tension even greater. At 9:00 a.m., I had to use the restroom, but I refused to leave that waiting room because I did not know what was going on behind those closed double doors. I elected to hold my urine because I refused to miss my name being called, allowing someone else who had just arrived to take my time slot.

Finally, through the side double doors that read Do Not Enter in bold red letters, a nurse emerged who called my name and told me to come on back. As I walked toward her, behind my back I gave Lew the thumbs-up—my way of telling him everything should go quickly once I got in the operating room.

That's exactly how it didn't go.

The nurse took me back to the same small room, told me to undress from the waist up, and to place my belongings in the plastic drawstring bag the hospital provided. *What? Not this again. Already been there, done that. What in the world is going on? Who is authorizing this?*

I cannot describe my distress and anguish as the technician took me back to that same room and took another 360° mammogram. This time it also included an ultrasound. When I complained about being given another mammogram, the nurse explained that another screening was done to know precisely where to inject the needle into the cyst to aspirate it.

This time the procedure was a little more bearable emotionally because I kept convincing myself it would all be over in a few minutes, then I would be on my way home. After holding my urine for so long, I asked if I could use the restroom. She told me it was located back in the lobby through the double doors.

I hurried through those doors, entering the lobby with my hospital gown held tightly closed. Lew looked up from his

9

smartphone and spotted me darting through the lobby. He thought the procedure was over because I had been in the back for such a long time. I assured him that from here everything should go as planned. With a quick wave to him, I headed back through those Do Not Enter doors.

Kind Words, Gentle Hands

The same nurse escorted me to a small operating room with various high-tech machines, gauze, needles, bandages, and the like. The operating room nurse introduced herself and helped me onto a table. She instructed me to lie down while she proceeded to go over the risks involved with the procedure, and she also shared with me the privacy HIPPA laws.

As I lay there, my heart raced. I had no words. I continued to pray silently. I asked God to guide the physician's hands, to allow him to see the cyst clearly so he could remove it in its entirety. I also prayed I would experience none of the risks the nurse had shared. My main prayer was "Please let this be my last procedure regarding my breast."

My refusal to speak was apparent. The attending nurse kept asking me, "Why are you so quiet?"

"I don't usually talk when I am going through something like this."

My main reason for being quiet was fear. I best conquer my fear through prayer and reflection. After all, someone was getting ready to plunge a huge needle into my breast, and I wanted to harness all the time I had to pray the doctor's hands were steady and that he would get all of the cyst out. I had suffered from intense breast pains for so long; I just wanted permanent and lasting relief.

As I lay there meditating and anticipating the surgery, what kept coming to mind was a question I had never asked myself or any other human being. These words played over in my mind like a song on repeat: "Why do I continually get cysts, and how can I rectify this?" The nurse wanted to keep talking to me, but recognizing I was in deep thought, she continued to prep me by sterilizing the entire breast, particularly the area where the aspiration was to take place, followed by getting the surgical tools ready for the doctor.

While she was prepping, the doctor walked in. He went right to the machine near me that had the picture of my breast and leaned in to get a closer look to see where he would begin. After closely examining the mammogram film, he warmly introduced himself, scrubbed and prepped, and proceeded to insert a huge needle into my breast to numb the area where the aspiration was to take place.

At that moment, I broke my silence and asked the nurse to please hold my hand. She gladly agreed. The nurse was quite kind. She was tender and caring in her approach. I could genuinely feel her love for what she does and for her patients. I no longer felt alone. Someone in the room cared about me. During the entire procedure, she comforted me. She continued to hold and rub my hand, and she kept asking, "Are you doing okay, sweetie?"

Her kind words put me at ease. Lying on that operating room table, I felt the love of God so strongly. His love always assures me that although I am going through these hard health challenges and I do not know what my future holds, I will be all right, whatever I face.

"Thank God, and Thank You, Doctor"

Amid the nurse's questions, the doctor interjected, "I got it all, and there's no need for another mammogram."

On the heels of his statement, I blurted out, "Thank God, and thank you, doctor."

As the nurse bandaged my breast and helped me into a sitting position, the doctor removed his gloves, turned to face me, looked me straight in the eyes, and shared a story that had taken place the night before. He said he heard the same words come from a sports player's mouth when he scored. "What does God have to do with any of this?" the doctor asked.

In that split second, as I sat in the semi-dark operating room, I waited for guidance from the Holy Spirit on how to answer respectfully. I was so elated everything was over, I did not want to mess up anything by the wrong words emanating from my mouth.

I wanted to be sure I spoke accurately and respectfully. I humbly responded, "Doctor, with all due respect, I do not know much about sports, so I cannot say why the sports player said what he said, but what I know for sure is that after suffering many years and having problems with my breasts, when you said you got it all and there was no need for a mammogram, your declaration created a knee-jerk response from me, and I'm so grateful to God for you and the success of what just took place for me today."

"That's Life"

The doctor seemed to hang on to my words for a minute, then he extended his hand toward mine. As we shook hands, he said, "It was nice meeting you," and something miraculous happened. While his hand gripped mine, I felt the energy shift in the room.

At the time, I was not sure if something changed because I was elated the procedure was over and he had extracted all of the cyst, or if it was the love of God I felt so strongly. Without thought or retrospect, I asked the doctor a question I had never asked any other medical professional. I asked the question I was pondering the entire time I was going through the operation. "Why do I continue to get cysts, and what can I do to stop getting them?"

He released my hand and turned around to go out the door. As he walked out, it seemed as if he was walking into another dimension. He left the dimly lit room and slowly walked down the brightly lit endless hallway with his white lab coat swaying behind him with each stride. As he transitioned from the dark to the light, he threw up his hands and said, "That's life, and there's nothing you can do about it."

I sat on the edge of the hospital bed almost in a trance and watched him disappear from my semi-lit room down the long, bright corridor. To my amazement, my ears clearly heard what he said, but my heart signaled to me that the answer I have long waited for was on the horizon. Was the doctor's response on point, or did my longing heart betray me?

Chapter Two

Years of Fear

We cannot direct the wind, but we can adjust the sails.[3]
~ Dolly Parton

One month later, the pain in my breast returned. For the first time in my life, I had enjoyed four weeks of freedom from pain, but the surgeon's words—"That's just a part of life"—continued to resound in my head. Although I could not bear the thought of it, I could not help but wonder if the return of pain indicated another cyst had formed. The first radiologist had warned me, "If a cyst develops more than three times in the same breast, then the next step would be to cut it out versus doing another aspiration."

The doctor who had performed the aspiration shared with me that too many aspirations and recurrences of cysts in the same breast indicated another method must be tried. The intensity of the pain made it nearly impossible to ignore. This was the kind of pain where nothing can bring relief. I tried warm compresses. When that failed, I let hot water from the shower run down my breast to ease the pain. It hurt to wear the most loose-fitting bra, and it was painful to lie on my stomach. The worst part was my instinctive cringe when Lew and my daughter, Mikayla, gently hugged me. Every time they came in for a hug, I threw up my arm to block them—a warning for them to pause so they would not unintentionally hug me too hard.

The pain was familiar, yet this time, it returned with a vengeance.

Kicking the Can down the Road

This type of unrelenting throbbing pain started in my sophomore year of college when I was nineteen years old and three hundred miles from home. My mom had moved to Eastern Shore, Virginia, and although she was closer than my home state of New Jersey, I did not want to go to an unfamiliar doctor or hospital near her. Familiarity has always been an added comfort to me.

I had no way or means of leaving college and flying back to New Jersey to seek medical attention. My college infirmary only handled minor incidents like an upset stomach, a headache, or a common cold. Its staff was not equipped to handle cases like mine.

Time passed and I kept kicking the can down the road before I got up the nerve to have a medical professional examine me to find out what was going on. I feared the worst. It was quite daunting that the pain hit me during October, the month that had been deemed Breast Cancer Awareness Month. It seemed as if every commercial played into my deepest fears. Unfortunately, DVRs had not yet been invented, so I could not ignore the situation by fast-forwarding the commercials and public service announcements. Younger generations do not realize how often women had to watch those frightening commercials.

Every time I was confronted with the slightest reminder something terrible could be going on in my breast, I trembled inside. When those commercials aired while I watched my 12-inch black-and-white television with my college roommate, I often got up from my bed and walked out of my dorm room, then returned after I physically counted down thirty or sixty seconds—the length of commercials at that time. I wanted to make sure that when I walked back into the room those scary commercials were not emanating from the television.

Unfortunately, the commercials did not stop. They were persistent. They kept coming. Seeing one consecutive cancer commercial after another made me wonder if the advertisements were a direct sign from God, informing me something was fatally wrong. Although I left my room often, my roommate did not suspect anything out of the ordinary, because it was common practice for teenagers to run to the restroom during commercials. Although she didn't notice my unusual behavior, I was not sure how long I could keep my secret.

Quite honestly, I was afraid to tell anyone because I was fighting an inner battle against fear and the negative thoughts that repeatedly bombarded me. If I shared this secret with anyone, I believed they would confirm what I was thinking, and I did not want negative words spoken over me or to me. Yes, at that young age, I knew the power of the spoken word. It wasn't just wishful thinking for me. I strongly believed that keeping a positive outlook would help me get through even the most difficult times. I even went so far as to think that positivity would help whatever was going on in my breast to heal on its own.

I was wrong.

Over time, I realized that no amount of wishful, positive thinking could make the pain go away. I have matured to know that positivity along with actions are the best formulas. But I pushed through anyway. I felt as if I had no other choice but to continue in school and let the chips fall where they may. At times, when the pain escalated, adverse thoughts ran rampant through my mind. Truthfully, I am not sure how I managed these overwhelming thoughts and emotions and still got through my studies to repeatedly make the Dean's List.

Regrettably, hiding my pain made it exponentially worse. I have learned I cannot conquer what I will not confront. The pain took on a life of its own. It reshaped and reconfigured who I was. Across my college campus, I was known as an outgoing, fun-loving person, always there to make people laugh or to share insights with those who were going through challenging times. I still tried to be that fun person because it is who I am, and the positivity helped take my mind off my problem.

Yet as time continued to advance, the severity of the pain progressed with it. I started to lose myself. I was not comfortable talking with anyone about such a personal problem. By that point, the pain was so severe that when I talked to anyone, a sharp pain hit me, and I involuntarily flinched.

Most asked, "Are you okay?"

"Yes, I'm good," I always answered.

Later, I would be upset because the very thing that I was trying not to bring attention to was leaking out. Sometimes I appeared shy to my friends and associates because I was afraid to look people in the eyes, fearing they would detect I was hiding a deep, dark secret. Matter of fact, the way some people looked at me shocked me because it seemed as if they were reading me like an open book, reluctant to say anything but waiting for me to share the news first.

The pain was unrelenting. I just wanted it to stop. When I was around others, I felt as if the energy from the pain radiated everywhere I went. It seemed obvious that people knew what I was going through.

Revealing My Secret

When I could no longer stand to keep my secret, I decided to break the news to my roommate, hoping that getting it out in the open would bring me a level of relief. I used her as a test to see how easy or difficult it would be to share with others. I pondered what she would say. How would she react to this kind of news? By that time, she had known me for two years, and I had only shared positive news with her.

After contemplating how to approach the subject, I determined to start by telling her, "My left breast is swollen and feels like a lump is in there." The moment I even thought to share with her, my heart raced uncontrollably. I broke out in a sweat, and I felt as if I was going to faint.

I waited until she was settled in the room, then I asked her if she had anything to do because I needed to share something important with her. After I told her everything, her reply was nowhere near what I had hoped for. To my dismay, she sounded as if she was a paid spokesperson for the frightening commercials I had been running away from for the past month. I know she spoke out of concern for me, but I could not bear the truth. Unequivocally, she was telling me to do the right thing. Her response was filled with wisdom, but it was not the feedback I hoped for. She emphatically urged me to go home and get my breast checked.

Having another young adult my age speak so firmly evoked even greater fear. I had hoped she would say, "Girl, you are too young. It's nothing." But she did not say that. Remember, she was the test to see if I would share my secret with others, and her response made me recoil. After that day, fear caused me to vow to keep silent about my pain and to let it play out on its own. Fortunately, my roommate respected me enough to wait for me to reintroduce the subject. From that day forward, she never brought it up again, and neither did I.

I proceeded with my life as usual, hiding and masking my pain yet quietly praying for healing because I was afraid to take the necessary action. The pain of what could be was greater than my reality. There was too much to think about: my studies, going to classes, leaving Virginia to fly back to New Jersey to get checked out, reporting my absences to my professor. Where would I begin, and what would be the outcome of my actions? I did not know what to do. All I could think of was how badly I wanted relief, how badly I wanted the pain to just go away and dissolve. These were hard decisions for a teenager all alone and far away from home. My greatest desire was an understanding adult to share my fears with. I believed a caring, responsible adult would not only empathize with me but also assist me in taking action to get the issue resolved and allay my fears.

Years of Fear

In hindsight, I can see how early in my formative years fear gripped me and kept me in its grasp for a very long time. I constantly hid the ills that plagued me because I did not know how to frame the sentence to articulate unusual happenings in my young body. When I did share with others the strange occurrences taking place in my body, the adults in my life did nothing about them, nor did they ask probing questions that would help me better explain these incidents. At a young age, how do you describe to your family that your body is feeling weird? I had no words for what I was experiencing. I felt sick all the time, I was always tired, and most importantly, the common sicknesses children my age could overcome in a few days bound me to my bed for weeks.

I believe that no one took my health issues seriously because I was a high-functioning sick person. In elementary school, I earned all A's—back then, they were all O's. I played and jumped like any other kid my age, and I did not look sick. But inside I was weak and listless. Even food did not increase my energy. I suffered alone.

These childhood experiences had indelibly etched on my mind that I should not keep telling people my problems if they did not hear my silent cries. I had to fight for myself. Subconsciously, I had already resolved that, like the illnesses prior to college, I did not need to share this event either, because I might get the same unsatisfactory response. Being hundreds of miles away at college made my decision easier. No one in my family was around. They did not physically see what I was going through. The only way they could possibly know is if I told them. When I called home from time to time, I only shared how my classes were going because that is all that they asked about. I grew up in an era when no one asked, "How are you doing?" They asked about events and situations but not about personal feelings. I grew up with the belief that no news is good news. So, everyone back home assumed everything was going fine. My family did not inquire about anything else; neither did I share it.

Test of Interest

I am uniquely sensitive and discerningly observant. I believe people only ask about what they really want to know or are interested in. If I wanted to share something meaningful to me, I carefully and precisely offered a taste of what I wanted to say, then I watched how they responded. If people did not react the way I thought they should, then I limited what I said. How they handled delicate information determined the depth of what I conveyed. Because I am a very sensitive person, I have always tested people to see how they manage what I share with them. I am not the type of person who talks just to hear myself talk. When I open up about profound things, I want a response in kind. I love to have fun, but I am also a deep thinker, always looking for my tribe of likeminded people.

I divulged only a little information at a time and then said to myself, "Let's see how they handle that." If people passed my unscientific test by showing genuine interest and giving solid, constructive advice, then I felt at ease and offered more details.

because it seemed to me that they were able to help me without making me feel regret for even bothering to share it. Oftentimes, I felt I was better off keeping things to myself because the pain of someone misunderstanding something I deemed too important and precious to divulge was a greater risk for me than just telling it. If people were halfhearted about what I told them, then they received increasingly less information from me, and our relationship was reduced to common courtesies like, "Hi, how are you?" and "How's the weather?" These niceties were safer for me than pouring out my heart to those who showed no passion for what I disclosed. With their mouths they said they were interested, but their actions showed otherwise.

I have always had a high level of intuition, even when I was much younger and did not know what discernment was. Over the years, I have grown to learn what it means to perceive beyond the spoken word. I have developed my divine gift by observing, paying close attention, and acting on what I have been given. I have learned not to ignore the energy I pick up from people. "When someone shows you who they are, believe them the first time."[4] I was so excited when I discovered this quote by Maya Angelou. Her words resonated with me, and they have stayed true and consistent. I have learned when and to whom to disclose sensitive information and when to keep it to myself. That knowledge has served me well and prevented a lot of heartache.

An "Invisible Illness"

To this day, I marvel how keenly aware I was at such a young age of how my body functioned. Of course, I could not explain what was going on, but nonetheless I knew something out of the ordinary was happening. I knew it instinctively and intuitively. As far back as I can remember, I knew my body was different from my siblings. I was the one who was often physically sick. Even when it did not show outwardly, I never really felt healthy internally. I went on with business as usual because I took my cues from those older than I was. To the best of my ability, I told them what I thought was going on in my body, but they seemed to show little to no concern. Their inaction led me to believe that maybe it

19

was just the way I was, and everything would be all right.

As far as my health is concerned, I feel as if I have never been heard. It took me forty-one years to learn that the medical profession calls this an "invisible illness"—a person looks fine outwardly, but inside their body's chronic illness and inflammation are wreaking havoc. One of the greatest telltale signs for me as a child was my incredibly low energy level. I always felt like I did not have enough breath to carry on with the slightest activities. True to form, I pushed on anyway. Therefore, no one seemed to notice my distress or difficulty. But I certainly felt it. When my classmates and I went out to play at recess, I was out of breath and tired by the time I ran out of the school building to the playground, which was not that far away. When I played with neighborhood children for any length of time, I felt physically sick to my stomach. One thing that stood out was needing to sit down and recoup after moderate exercise, whereas others my age who participated in the same exercises were fully energized and ready to play even harder.

My girth was also disproportionate to the rest of my small frame. Even when I first woke up, without having anything to eat or drink, my stomach protruded. I also suffered from acne and scarring long before puberty started for me. My mom did take note of that, so she boiled water and added boric acid to it, then washed my face at night, hoping the treatment would clear up my acne. Reflecting on those childhood issues confirms these were all telltale signs of ensuing bigger ones that may have turned out differently had they been handled differently.

Going with the Flow

Fortunately, despite not getting the help I so desperately needed, I seemingly survived it all, even the lump in my breast and the debilitating pain. I kept going with the flow of life. My sophomore year in college ended, and I went home for the summer and slept almost the entire summer away. I told no one about the pain. Before I knew it, two more years had passed, and I graduated with honors, still dealing with the fact that something was going on in my breast and my entire body.

Once graduation was behind me, I had a clear sense of accomplishment. I believed that one compartmentalized event in my life was over, and I could clearly think about what I needed to do before I started my career.

Juggling too many things always got the best of me. Constant sickness, tiredness, and just never feeling quite my best were all telltale signs leading up to my greatest discovery. I searched for a primary care physician and found one who could fit me in on my time schedule. In her office, I probably told her way more than she could bear to hear. I poured out my heart about how long I had suffered; I shared with her the pain and the fear of what might be going on. She hinted I might have a cyst.

Growing up, I never heard about a cyst. Anytime I heard about a lump of any kind, cancer was associated with it. Had I heard the word *cyst*, I could have been thinking differently all along. After listening to my story and examining me, she observed that my breast was swollen. But to my surprise, she said I was too young to have a mammogram. On that day, I learned mammograms have an age limit. She did not even do an ultrasound. She did a physical exam and said she did not detect a lump. She then advised me to do self-exams and keep an eye on any unusual events. She also said, "If the pain worsens or any other changes occur, then schedule an appointment right away to see me and let me know."

With her findings, I asked myself, "Did I get the miracle I have been praying for?" I was elated that nothing out of the ordinary was found. Her advice gave me unspeakable joy. Another adult, but this time a licensed medical doctor was not worried, so why should I be?

Pursing an Answer

But the pain worsened and became extremely intolerable. I wanted a doctor who would perform an ultrasound to see what was really going on. "Something is there, and I know it," I told myself. I wanted to see the best doctor possible, so I sought recommendations from family and friends. By this time, I was doggedly pursuing an answer. The pain had gone on way too long.

I questioned other females in my life to see if they had also experienced this type of pain in their breasts. Every female I spoke to assured me that my situation was not normal. They expressed that once a month during their menstrual cycle, they might feel slight discomfort or tenderness in their breasts, but nothing compared to what I had been complaining about.

Armed with this knowledge, I became adamant about getting to the root cause. I was compelled to find another doctor who would do the tests I felt that I needed. One friend recommended an obstetrician/gynecologist (OBGYN), a doctor who specifically deals with educating female patients about disease prevention and early detection of diseases that affect reproductive health.

The search continued for years. After Lew and I became engaged, I did not want to bring this old pain into my new marital relationship. I wanted a fresh start in life and with Lew. I had already suffered for eight years, wondering how to get some relief and was more than ready for all of this to be behind me.

I called the office of the OBGYN that my friend recommended. When the nurse answered the phone, I told her all I had been through and how scared I was. She attentively listened to what I said and assured me it was normal to feel afraid given the circumstances. She also confirmed that this doctor and his staff would take very good care of me. Her voice and her words comforted and reassured me. With that level of kindness on display, I knew this was the doctor for me. Remember, I am an empath and pick up other people's unspoken and spoken energy. She asked if I was ready to schedule an appointment and I said, "Yes, let's do it."

The Best Listener

I met with the doctor, and as I had done with the nurse, I told him everything about my health history and how I had noticed that I am different from other people. "I am always tired, and my left breast really hurts and has been swollen since I was nineteen years old."

What stood out so vividly to me was that he was the best listener. As I spoke, he exhibited a lot of care and concern, as if I were his very own daughter. When I spoke about the pain, his reaction was not stoic; he flinched at each description. Everything—and I mean everything—I had held back for years was unleashed on this caring doctor.

He said he was going to examine me and asked me to lie down on the examining table. Before he proceeded with the examination, he called the attending nurse into the room with him, and once he started to probe around my swollen breast, he ordered a mammogram immediately. I was in utter shock that something was finally going to be done, even though I had been told I was too young for a mammogram.

Other doctors never seemed to listen to me at the point that I needed them the most. I know there are protocols to follow, but listening to what a patient has to say about her body should be tantamount. No one knows my body the way I do. After all, I live in my body 24/7. I'm aware if something does not feel right even if I do not have a medical test to corroborate what I am experiencing. Fortunately, this new doctor took what I shared with him seriously. His listening acumen and bedside manner were so comforting.

A Pink Rose

The nurse came and escorted me to another room, where I would wait until the mammogram was administered. Within that room was a small opening with a privacy curtain. It housed a vertical locker with a key to place all my belongings in. The outer waiting room was beautifully decorated with high-end furnishings and plush carpeting. Every magazine imaginable was lying on the tables. The nurse, the doctor, and the atmosphere made me feel well cared for and special.

After I had my mammogram, I was escorted back to this posh waiting room while the film was being read. The wait felt quite long. Once they were ready for me, the nurse called me back into the room, where the doctor would come and share his findings. Eventually, I heard a slight knock on the door, then the door opened, and my doctor came into the room to speak with me. But this time he was accompanied by three more doctors.

My heart skipped a beat.

"Oh my gosh, did they wait too late to test me?" I asked myself.

Four doctors in white coats looking at me made the situation seem very serious. My doctor sat down next to me and took me by the hand and said, "A lump was found and with your permission, I would like to proceed with an ultrasound to determine the nature of it."

"Yes, by all means. Can we do it right now?"

I was beyond ecstatic something was finally being done with such care and precision. Within the next hour, the ultrasound was performed, and the lump was a cyst. I asked the doctor, "Can you take it out right now?"

He chuckled, then said, "No these things have to be scheduled."

He gave me the number to the scheduler's office and explained the procedure, informing me of what I could expect when they went in and removed the cyst. I was totally fine with everything he shared because of the way he treated me. I had total confidence he would be sure everything would go as planned.

I later learned the other three doctors were doctors in training. The nurse escorted me back to the room where my belongings were housed in a locker to get dressed, and when I was fully dressed, she walked with me back through the waiting room area that leads to the lobby. As I was leaving the waiting room and headed to the lobby area, a nurse at the kiosk handed me a pink rose and said she would see me soon. I said to myself, "What a special touch to be given a rose after having a mammogram."

A Dark Cloud Lifts

Although what I experienced was terrifying, the care that I felt at this New Jersey Breast Center made it bearable. They seemed to care about me as a whole person, and I genuinely felt their concern. When I arrived at my car, I replayed all I had just experienced. I decided not to go directly to my apartment alone but rather took a detour to my sister Charlene's house to let her know what I had suspected all along was indeed true.

After I arrived at her home, I rang her doorbell. When Charlene opened the door, I was so overwhelmed with emotion that I had braved such news by myself that as soon as I saw her face I immediately fell into her arms and told her, "They found a lump." I distinctly remember the horror on her face. I kept saying repeatedly, "I knew something was wrong for years, but it seemed as if no one was listening to me until now." She helped me into her house and listened to me rehash all that had transpired. Before leaving to go home, she prayed with me and continued to tell me she believed I would come through this.

Days later, the cyst was removed, and the Breast Center sent it to the lab for further testing. I was sent home with explicit instructions for caring for the place where they had removed the cyst. A week later, I received a letter in the mail, letting me know that the lab report found the cyst to be benign.

That was the happiest day of my life.

Finally, my worst fears were put to rest. I could get on with my life and get married without the fear I had faced day in and day out for years. I felt as if I had been given a new lease on life. The dark cloud of doom had seemingly lifted, and I could hardly wait to get on with the business of living.

Chapter Three

Lifestyle Changes

The wish for healing has always been half of health.[5]
~ Lucius Annaeus Seneca

The small glimpses of joy I received from having cysts removed from my breast and getting some relief from pain was the impetus that compelled me to go whole hog regarding my health. Unbeknownst to me, though, cysts in my breast were only a manifestation of a greater problem. Although I wanted to push the Pause button and take a rest from it all, I had to courageously forge ahead, even though I did not know my next step.

I had always wanted to know what it was like to live a healthy, vibrant life. It seemed as if everyone in my circle was afforded this awesome gift except me. Don't get me wrong. I was never bitter or upset; I was just curious as to why I was so sickly. I repeatedly pondered why I never had a chance to experience complete health. In trying to make sense of it all, I shared these thoughts frequently with my mom, hoping she would have the answer I longed for.

After much questioning, she too desperately wanted to find the answers I searched for. She oftentimes speculated and repeatedly said, "You are probably going through these things because before I had you, I had an ectopic pregnancy, or maybe because I only had one fallopian tube when you were born, or probably because I had you when I was going through the change of life." All of those things may have been valid, but neither one of us knew for certain. In times of self-reflection, over and over I envisioned myself healed. I could not fathom going through my entire life repeatedly sick.

No Viable Solutions

To move forward in my beliefs, I sought out help beyond what I could offer myself. I was at an impasse, though. No matter what method I tried, I made no progress. I searched for professionals who, after lengthy conversations about my health challenges, assured me they had the answer to help me. But when I sat in their office to talk about the details of my symptoms, they could never come up with a viable solution. Every year, medical testing and screening once again proved I was not getting better but growing progressively worse.

Everything spiraled so quickly; I literally had no time to breathe. My first diagnosis was breast cysts. The next one was chronic anemia. After that diagnosis was amenorrhea and following that was high cholesterol. Can you imagine? Every year I went for my checkup only to be told that the lab reports showed something new, something different. Before I processed one diagnosis, another one came that, in my mind, was even worse than the previous one.

This was too much for my twenty-something self to handle. *Why am I having all these symptoms at such a young age, and how can I fix my body to eliminate these things?* With the diagnosis of high cholesterol, I reached a point of wondering why I went to the doctor's office to keep getting a negative report with no help offered that I felt was sustainable. Taking an iron pill and Provera and birth control pills did nothing for my body. The iron pills didn't raise my heme iron levels, taking Provera and birth control pills did not cause my menstruation to return to normal. Over time, my lab results did not budge. I was broken physically and emotionally.

Not intending to be rude, I one day said to my doctor, "It's a shame that my symptoms are progressing, and new ones are cropping up, and I'm continuously getting worse on your watch." I was so frustrated by getting yearly checkups only to be told each time I was deteriorating. He seemed perplexed by my statement, but he never offered any further suggestions or comments.

With each passing year, I could not help but ask myself, "Will I be totally healed on this side of eternity?" I know going to heaven is the ultimate healing, but I longed to experience a day without sickness, disease, and pain in this life.

A Radical Lifestyle Choice

With little to no help or answers from the medical field, I decided to try something different to take my life back and have some control over the gloomy outcomes. At that time, over thirty years ago, Lew and I, in our quest to live a healthier lifestyle, sat down to figure out what we could do together to help me achieve my health goals. We were already riding our bikes daily in and around our neighborhood, but he felt we should try something else. He strongly encouraged me to believe that we would see results if we employed other measures in addition to riding our bikes, so the next day we began another form of exercise.

We started off by taking long walks on the trails in our beautiful, expansive county park replete with playgrounds, walking and running trails, tennis courts, sports fields, and archery ranges. Walking in this picturesque park was a daily adventure. We met so many wonderful people who were there for the same reason—to enjoy the view while they exercised. I loved being around like-minded people who also wanted to improve their health.

Walking in the park daily was going so well we looked into other things we could do to facilitate and enjoy a healthy lifestyle. Our next venture was so radical some of our family members laughed and shook their heads when Lew and I announced we were going to eat only organic foods. No more preservatives, pesticides, and ingredients we could not pronounce or understand. This decision was huge! Back in the early nineties, we didn't know anyone else who purchased all organic foods. We were not trying to be bougie. We were just longing to do whatever we could to be healthier.

In the meantime, I continued to go for my annual medical screenings, but even with all the changes I made, the results still showed no change. "None of this makes sense," I told myself. "What could possibly be wrong with me? I'm working out every day, and I'm eating very healthy, but the health needle is not moving in my favor."

I tried to get my mind off the results and focus solely on the fact that I was doing everything I knew to do. Maybe if I stayed steadfast, something would eventually change, and I would get the breakthrough I had worked for, so I centered more on what brought me pleasure than on my pain and suffering.

My favorite part of embarking on a healthy lifestyle was that I unquestionably enjoyed the workouts in the park. They gave me such an adrenaline rush that I wanted to walk seven days a week, rain or shine. Although I did not notice any changes in my health by incorporating the organic foods I ate, exercise played a major role in my emotional health. Each day I walked, I felt more invigorated and at peace. The longer I walked, the better I felt. Lew and I started out by doing one lap on the trail, and we worked our way up to three laps, including a steep hill. After a while, we moved so quickly that athletes in the park tried to keep up with us.

Pay Now or Pay Later

I truly believed that if I was getting fit, then I was getting healthier, but my new lab results still showed no change. I then began to question the validity of eating strictly organic foods. I wanted to see some results for my efforts, and the high cost of organic foods with no medical changes in sight was so discouraging. We often shopped for groceries twice a week to restock our refrigerator. I regularly asked Lew, "How are we going to continue to shop at this 'whole paycheck' store? Is buying organic really worth it?"

He continued to reassure me. "Although the needle on your health doesn't seem to be moving, eating this way will reward you in the long run." He added, "Either you pay now, or you will pay later."

I didn't want to pay later. With my fragile health, I did not want to go back to eating conventional foods grown with pesticides and herbicides. But I also wanted to ensure we could continue to afford to eat organically grown food in the years to come. If we had to go back to conventional food due to our budget, it would be a great setback for me. I had to move forward with momentum to give my body time to prove to me it was doing better with the new food and exercise, even though my test results said otherwise.

Like Lew, I hoped I was moving in the right direction, so I decided to not worry about the cost and instead focus on the fact that I was getting healthier by eating well and exercising. "One day," I told myself, "my blood results will match up with what I'm doing. I am doing a good thing for my body, and that is all I should be concerned about." However, in the back of my mind, I often wondered why I was not seeing the results I thought I should see. I was eating 100-percent organic foods and exercising every day. Surely something should be different. One part of me was happy to know I was doing something great for myself, but that elation was short-lived because my goals were not being realized.

The Back Label

It took years for me to learn that eating 100-percent organic foods does not guarantee they are 100-percent healthy for me. I purchased everything I enjoyed eating as long as it was labeled organic. Armed with even greater knowledge now, I have become a wiser shopper and have discarded that type of thinking. Everything labeled organic was not good for me. I learned the hard way, and I paid a hefty price for that lack of knowledge. Once I learned to read labels, I became a savvy shopper. All food is not equal. Some organic foods can be highly processed and include added ingredients. I no longer read only the front label. I also read the ingredients on the back.

Unbeknownst to me, the other ingredients on the back label were wreaking havoc on my body. I did not know there were harmful ingredients in the foods I purchased because I was only reading the front labels. I had to train myself to read the labels on the back to be sure the other ingredients were safe for me to consume. Today I am an avid label reader, and if there is anything on the label I do not understand or cannot pronounce, I will not purchase that product. Reading labels has been a game-changer on my road to health and wellness, and I have trained Lew and Mikayla to read the back labels also because we are Team Dawn when it comes to my health.

Years of following a strict regimen and still not seeing the desired health results was disconcerting. I have always been solution driven. I can survive practically anything if I know there is a reason and a solution. In addition to diversifying my exercise, eating organic was a step in the right direction. I spent hours in the supermarket reading the labels of everything I planned on purchasing. Reading each label gave me some assurance I was getting what I was paying for. Organic food can be quite expensive, and I want my money to be well spent.

Long term, I wanted to see different results in my blood work report. As an immediate result, I hoped to alleviate my daily pain. I have never masked my pain; therefore, I was acutely aware when pain came and when it left. My top priority was to seek out a remedy, not just dull the pain. Therefore, over-the-counter medicines were out of the question. I wanted to get to the root cause of why the pain occurred in the first place. Pain is my body's signal something is wrong. Pain relievers can numb the pain, but they do not solve the problem of the pain. I choose to suffer through the pain until I can get to the reason the pain exists.

A Welcome Alternative

A while after my breast aspiration, I was jolted out of my sleep by a stabbing pain in my left breast. Sitting straight up in bed so suddenly, I startled Lew, who was lying next to me. He immediately thought I was having a bad dream. I told him that a sharp pain in my breast woke me out of my sleep. As I clutched my breast, hoping to ease the pain, I continued to scream.

Lew tried to reassure me. "It could be phantom pains. That usually happens after an invasive procedure." After he had hernia surgery when he was a little boy, the pain came back for years, even into adulthood, as if the hernia had returned. His words brought me some comfort, but I knew deep down inside it was imperative for me to find out what was going on.

A month prior, I had had a mammogram and another breast aspiration. I thought having another mammogram would be way too soon. My concern was that frequent mammograms may subject me to excessive radiation exposure my body was not able to detoxify. During one of my many blood tests, I was also diagnosed with Non-Alcoholic Fatty Liver Disease (NAFLD). More health concerns arose when I knew my liver was compromised and could not get rid of the radiation like it would in a person with normal liver function. Finding the source of this pain seemed urgent, but I did not know how to do that without having another mammogram.

Not knowing exactly what to do, I decided to conduct an internet search on "Alternatives to Mammograms." To my surprise, the results yielded other choices I was not aware of. "Why haven't I heard about these alternatives, especially since I've had long-term breast issues?" I asked myself. After reading a few of the choices from the top of the list, the one that appealed to me the most was thermography. I decided to give it a try.

One of the best lessons I learned from discovering the first breast lump in my college years was the importance of quickly getting medical help to put my fears to rest so I did not suffer needlessly like I did at the tender age of nineteen. So, as soon as I learned about thermography, I dialed the local number provided on the web page and scheduled my first thermogram.

"Is That It?"

During the phone call, the nurse responsible for administering the thermograms shared extensively what I should expect. Since I always had breasts that hurt, I was elated to learn thermograms were totally different than mammograms. From her description, I concluded this was unmistakably going to be the best choice for me. The screening process emphatically put my mind at ease. The nurse explained, "Thermograms use infrared technology to determine changes in your breast long before they occur."

During my first appointment, the same registered nurse I had spoken to over the phone went over the entire procedure again in greater detail. Afterward, she had me undress from the waist up and told me to sit in a chair facing her while she used an infrared camera to take pictures of each breast. The infrared camera detects heat patterns and blood flow in the breast tissue. The results are then digitally produced and read by a medical doctor who is trained and certified to read the images and make a diagnosis. The entire process was quick and painless.

When my thermogram was completed, I could hardly believe how easy and pain free the experience was. In sheer disbelief, but utter joy, I repeatedly asked, "Is that it? Am I done?"

"That's all there is to this," responded the nurse. She then exited the room so I could get dressed in privacy.

That day, I left the thermography office with a song in my heart and a giddy pep in my step. Not having my tender breasts pulled and tugged and then smashed between plexiglass was so refreshing for me. On the long drive home, I said to myself, "This type of screening will allow my breast to finally have a chance to really heal."

A Shocking Realization

Before the thermogram was administered, I filled out extensive paperwork. One of the questions that was very enlightening to me was "How many mammograms have you had?" When I calculated the number in my mind by going back to my first one up until that point, the revelation left me in complete shock—thirty mammograms. I had never calculated the number because no one had ever asked me that question. Every time a lump was found, I had a mammogram to determine the nature of the lump.

To my knowledge, most people do not have that many mammograms in a lifetime. Dazed, I sat in the dimly lit office, reeling from the discovery I had suffered through so many of these procedures. In a split second, I knew that moving forward I would have to do something different. If I continued with this type of screening, my yearly exams would add at least seventy more mammograms, especially since I plan on living a long, healthy life. Having issues with my breasts since my college days has forced me to get mammogram screenings at a younger age than was recommended.

"The FDA approved thermography as an adjunctive tool in the assessment of breast masses in 1982."[6] Ironically, thermograms were approved by the FDA the same year I found the first lump in my breast. But I was not aware of this type of screening then, so I had to go with the one I knew was available, the one that is widely promoted. If I had known about this alternative screening in college, I could have gotten my results earlier than I did. Mammograms are typically recommended to women for the first time at age forty, whereas thermograms can be given at half that age.

I now choose thermograms as my first go-to method of screening, even though most conventional doctors do not acknowledge them or accept the report. I still do them for my sanity and peace of mind because I like knowing I can have screenings done that allow me to have full body autonomy. I enjoy having choices, so I am very happy with my decision.

Benefits of Dry Brushing

At that first appointment, when the nurse came back in the examining room to tell me that she would call me after the doctor read the images, she asked if I had ever done dry brushing. The week prior, I had fortuitously stumbled on an article about the benefits of dry brushing. I could hardly believe what I was hearing. Her question was another sign I was on my road to healing. I told her, "I use a body brush in the shower, but I have never dry brushed."

She shared the difference of brushing in the shower versus dry brushing. She told me, "Dry brushing helps to move your lymphatic system, and it will aid greatly in alleviating the pain in your breast."

That news excited me. If anyone needed to move pain out of the breast, it was me. That day I bought two dry brushes. When I arrived home, I researched everything I could find on the benefits of dry brushing. I discovered it is one method used to help move one of the most important systems in my body: the lymphatic system. I started dry brushing that day and have been dry brushing ever since. It is so invigorating. After a session of dry brushing, I feel awakened, refreshed, and less tense. Every day I faithfully dry brush starting from my toes to the top of my head. My goal is to use dry brushing as one method to help move all the stagnation from my lymph system. The nurse who does my thermograms is fully aware of the challenges I've had with my breast. Therefore, she encourages me to gently dry brush my breast to be sure the lymph is moving there also.

A Pea-Size Lump

After a year of dry brushing my entire body, I was standing in front of the mirror ready to begin my daily ritual of dry brushing. What I saw next startled me. I ran from my bathroom mirror to my full body mirror in my bedroom closet. I wanted to make certain what I was seeing was accurate, not just a shadow from the lighting. A pea-size lump protruded from my left breast.

After careful examination, I yelled downstairs for Lew to come upstairs to our master bathroom to take a look and confirm he could see exactly what I saw. When he told me he saw the same thing, I panicked. My heart raced, and I became very nervous and jittery. My mouth became extremely dry, and no amount of water could quench my thirst. Every other lump in my breast had been found because of intense pain. However, this one came without warning. One morning it was not there, and the next morning it was protruding from my skin. My emotions fluctuated between panic and shock. I did not want to believe what I saw in the mirror. That whole day, I watched the lump incessantly.

Months prior, when I had a thermogram, the nurse said cancer could be detected years before a lump develops because the thermogram picks up the slightest heat and can detect extra blood supply to that area. I kept repeating her words throughout the day. Was this some fluke? How did this happen? Once again fear reared his ugly head, and this time brought his big brother doubt with him. I was scared beyond measure.

I immediately called my OBGYN and told her what I had discovered. On June 8, 2017, I had an emergency doctor's appointment. I knew from past experience she would suggest a mammogram; therefore, I called ahead of time to let the doctor know I had found a visible lump, and therefore, there was no need for a mammogram. "If I can see it with the naked eye, then I do not need a machine to see it." I reiterated, "I have been recently diagnosed with liver disease and cannot have a mammogram because my liver cannot process the radiation." I then added, "I feel I am starting to gain momentum toward the road to healing; therefore, I do not want any setbacks."

They gave no indication they were unwilling to observe my wishes.

A Hard-Won Compromise

When I arrived, my doctor thoroughly examined me. Not only could she feel the lump, she said she could also see the lump. But to my dismay, she had already scheduled my mammogram before I got there. I pleaded with her to give me an ultrasound since the lump had already been found. "The purpose of the mammogram is to find a lump, isn't that correct?" I asked. We went back and forth as to why my health could not endure another mammogram, and she insisted no doctor would see me without one.

The tension was so strong in the room that I began to cry. I did not feel heard. It seemed that medical protocol trumped my needs and wishes. I could not wrap my mind around why I could not oversee my own health and get only the services I desired.

The doctor and I continued our dialogue as to why I was not a good candidate for a mammogram. For a while, neither of us budged on our stance, but we finally came to a compromise. Clearly, I had a lump that needed to be further examined, and the first step for medical science to check a breast lump is through a mammogram. I mustered the strength to ask my doctor to cancel the appointment at the hospital and send me instead to a private practice that uses less radiation. Above all else, I had to be an advocate for my own health. Thankfully, she agreed and made the necessary phone calls. The nurse in the doctor's office was also able to locate a private practice that specializes in mammography.

Much-Needed TLC

The day of the appointment, with medical records in hand, I arrived at the facility and explained my entire story and medical history to the receptionist who signed me in. Everyone was exceptionally kind—the receptionist, the scheduler, and the nurses. Each one was very caring and understanding. When I explained my fears, they did everything they could to let me know they would take extra care with me. I was so elated I had insisted on going to a private practice versus having the procedure at the hospital.

The whole atmosphere seemed more personal and less sterile. When it was time for the mammogram, the technician used every precaution to ensure she did not induce more pain. There must have been less pressure placed on the compressor because although I was in excruciating pain, I did not feel any additional pain from the equipment. The technician who administered the mammogram informed me that their facility had the lowest radiation numbers in the state. She said, "The radiation from our machines equals the radiation you will be exposed to on a short airplane ride." I was very relieved to hear this good news.

After the screening, I was escorted to a waiting room while the film was read. Finally, my name was called. As I took my seat in front of the computer monitors, I watched closely as the doctor read the film. It seemed as if the doctor took a long time to read the results. In my presence, he looked at the film over and over again.

There's nothing as frustrating as wanting an answer right away but having to wait for what feels like eternity. During this lengthy time, I began to shake uncontrollably, hoping for the best but thinking the worst. I could not turn off the negativity in my mind. I was out of control. I prayed, I meditated, and I even spoke positive affirmations under my breath, all to no avail. My body continued to shake in fear.

The radiologist, who also owned the breast center, commented on how nervous I was. When he read the film, he said the mammography did detect a lump, and he wanted to monitor it for three months to make sure there were no changes.

"What type of lump is it?" I asked.

"A fibrocystic lump, and I want to keep an eye on it for any abnormal changes." He then showed me how to do breast self-exams to detect any changes within that time frame. He also said, "If you notice anything out of the ordinary, call this office right away." Afterward, he escorted me back to the waiting area to schedule my three-month appointment.

An Unexpected Result

While I waited for my three-month checkup, I continued to dry brush and made sure to carefully dry brush around my left breast where the lump was discovered. I continued to check every day, as I was directed, to be sure there were no changes. Within the second month, I could no longer visibly see the lump; neither could it be detected through my self-exam.

Three months of waiting seemed like forever. When the day of my appointment finally arrived, I was eager to go and ready to get my clean bill of health. This was the first time a lump had been found, and the radiologist had not seen the need to have it removed.

At this examination, I was only given an ultrasound, not another mammogram. The technician checked my breast for over an hour. "What in the world could she be looking for?" I muttered to myself. *Please tell me what's going on.*

The technician was very quiet and focused. She continued to search my breast like she was looking for lost treasure. The procedure went on and on. She left the room several times, as if she were going to consult someone. When she returned, she had to continuously apply lubricant as she ran that scanner from my armpit to my nipple looking for the lump I was supposed to keep an eye on.

With each passing moment, my fear increased. I was so nervous that my body temperature dropped extremely low, and she offered me a blanket because she noticed I was shivering. The temperature in the room was approximately 70 degrees, but it felt like it was 20 degrees. As she handed me a second blanket, she said, "I'll be back. I have to get the doctor."

As she rushed out of the room, I hollered within myself, "What have you found? Please do not leave me here like this! Don't you know that you are scaring me? Why do you have to be so secretive? Just tell me what you have found!"

A few minutes later, she returned to the room with the doctor. Without saying a word to me, he also took the scanner, applied lubricant to it, and repeatedly scanned from my armpit to my nipple looking for the lump. After four or five passes, he handed the scanner back to the nurse and told her to have me get dressed and meet him in his office.

"In your office? I get to bypass the waiting room this time. Oh God, this is serious!" I muttered.

After I dressed and took a seat in his office, he reprimanded me for letting my nerves get the best of me before he gave me the results. He said, "You need to calm down and stop being so nervous."

"I have been through a lot in the past fifteen years," I said, "and nothing seems to have let up or given me a break. In 2015, I was diagnosed with five autoimmune diseases. Therefore, everything that happens to me is just another straw that breaks the proverbial camel's back." I added, "It's not the things that happen here or there, but it is a culmination of events that have made me such an emotional wreck. I do not want to be nervous or live in fear, but I have been caught up in the web of bad news regarding my health."

When I finished speaking, he said, "Well, the ultrasound shows the cyst is gone."

Before the final words left his lips, the biggest and brightest smile spread across my face.

He went on to say, "I won't need to see you again until your next yearly exam."

The Biggest Smile in the Waiting Room

Those words were music to my ears. A huge weight dropped off my shoulders. I walked into that waiting room with a pep in my step I hadn't had in quite some time. When I arrived at the waiting room entrance that leads to the lobby, I scanned the people in the lobby looking for some friendly face I could flash a smile to. I just wanted to let someone know how happy I was that I was going to be okay. Fear had gripped me for three months, and I had been freed from its stronghold.

As I panned the waiting room of about a dozen women waiting in the lobby for their annual screening, I could not find one who appeared friendly enough to smile at. I was so excited about my news that I searched the room one more time, and lo and behold, I found the brightest angelic face with a smile was so big I thought I was seeing a mirage. I had to do a double take.

Wait a minute. This cannot be real. Oh my goodness.

"Hey, what are you doing here?"

The person with the biggest smile happened to be Lew. He showed up without telling me because he wanted to be sure that when I walked out of the doctor's office, he was there to support me with whatever news I had received. I guess he could tell from the smile on my face that I had received a favorable report.

We walked hand in hand as he escorted me to my car. He opened the driver side of the car to let me in first, and when he came around and sat in the passenger seat, we embraced. I held him tightly, not ever wanting to let him go as I cried tears of joy and relief. On the drive home, my mind swirled as I wondered how my breast had escalated from cysts that can be aspirated to a fibrocystic breast.

Chapter Four

A Long, Arduous Process

If someone wishes for good health, one must first ask oneself if he is ready to do away with the reasons for his illness. Only then is it possible to help him.[7]

~ **Hippocrates**

I vividly remember when I first heard the medical term *tipping point*. At that precise moment, everything I had gone through in my health made total sense. With each doctor's visit, something else was always found. No matter how hard I worked to be healthy, some other unexplainable issue presented itself either in my blood work or on a mammogram. But the moment I was exposed to that term, I repeatedly saw it or heard holistic healers talk about it. Hearing the term was another signpost pointing the way, letting me know I was on the right track. The biblical principle of "seek and you will find" was in full play, for sure (Matthew 7:7 NIV).

The tipping point occurred when my toxicity load got so heavy it created a major health crisis.[8] It didn't happen suddenly; it was building one sickness at a time. This clearly explained why I was not seeing the results I longed for from my blood work, and it also clarified why I always felt so ill. The health crisis I experienced crept up on me layer upon layer until my body could not take it anymore. Tipping point also explains why every time I went to the doctor I was getting worse not better, because the root cause of my sickliness was not being addressed. The symptoms were being treated, not the cause.

A Team of Experts

Each year when I went for my annual checkups, my blood test showed I was getting progressively worse. I took the results of my lab tests very seriously, so I never ignored the outcome. However, by nature I am one who perseveres. I do not let what's happening to me get the best of me. Therefore, I never quit trying. I kept eating healthy, exercising, and going for my annual doctor visits. I was dismayed by the huge roadblock to getting to the root cause of my issue, but I also knew that, despite it all, I had to keep doing everything I knew to do and stay steadfast to living my life the best I could until the answer came. Having a loving husband who supports me wholeheartedly is also a tremendous help. Despite how sick I became, nothing on the outside changed. I still was a great wife to Lew, a wonderful mother to Mikayla, a productive employee to my employer, and I was even diligent to contributing time and resources to my local church.

To the undiscerning eye, everything looked fine, but I felt like I was literally dying inside. From New Jersey to Virginia, I sought out the collective wisdom of medical doctors, naturopathic doctors, holistic doctors, herbalists, chiropractors, and iridologists. I believe that one person cannot have all the answers and that en masse we could come up with the root-cause answer to my problem. I needed a squad who could peel back the layers of my intricate being and unearth exactly what was going on in the deep recesses of my inner parts all the way down to the cellular level. Consequently, I gathered a team of experts whom I hoped could put the puzzle pieces together so I could see the total picture of who I am and what is happening inside my body.

I went to never-ending lengths to try to get to the root cause. I spared no expense. My health is important, and I am willing to invest in it at any cost. Over the years, my life savings plummeted, and my energy reserves diminished. Yet I kept pouring more of my earnings into resources I thought would help me find a way to heal and get better so I could live a happy, healthy, vibrant life.

It has always been health over money. I told myself, "When I feel better and am healed, I will be able to earn the money back that I've invested on my health." I innately knew optimal health would make life more enjoyable. Health is wealth, and having a whole body would free up precious time I spent searching for health. Being free from sickness would afford me the time and energy to generate all the revenue I need.

Enlisting the help of many experts meant more testing, more paperwork, more questioning, and more money. Traveling from one appointment to another, talking with one professional after another, rehashing and restating my life history and health symptoms became physically and mentally draining. Worst of all, at the end of each meeting, writing that check and still having no answers left me feeling mentally destitute and financially depleted.

What's Missing?

I always sensed some critical step was missing. These appointments seemed all too familiar, albeit with different experts. My mind kept telling me something in my medical history should have set off alarms, prompting my team to probe for further action.

I related my full medical history at each appointment. My mother birthed me, her seventh child, at the age of thirty-three, and afterward her menstrual cycle never returned. I was a weak and sickly child and still felt that way. My menstrual cycle started at age thirteen but did not return until my sophomore year in high school. From middle school through college, I was a gymnast, so my sporadic menstrual cycle was attributed to excessive exercise. However, after I graduated from college, my menstrual cycle was still irregular. When I returned to my home state, my resolve was renewed to continue my fight. Therefore, I was relentless in sharing the quirky things occurring in my body regardless of how exasperating it could be.

Finally, my OBGYN had another series of tests done, and I was diagnosed with secondary amenorrhea and prescribed birth control pills to help restart my menstrual cycle. "Amenorrhea is the absence of menstruation, often defined as missing one or more missed menstrual periods. Secondary amenorrhea refers to the absence of three or more periods in a row by someone who has had periods in the past."[9] Within six months of being on the pill, my cycle still did not restart; therefore, I was given a script for Provera with the hopes that this medication would induce my menstrual cycle. Each medical expert I consulted heard all these facts.

Laboring to find the root cause allowed fatigue to creep in, but my determination to continue fighting grew stronger. I could not succumb to this weight of despair. Giving up was never an option. I had too much on the line to lose. Copious amounts of my time and resources had already been invested, so I carried on with the process. The methods I had tried in the past did not work. Therefore, I wanted a different path.

Albert Einstein is accredited with saying, "The definition of insanity is doing the same thing over and over again but expecting different results."[10] Each expert had his or her own theory of how to make my blood work look different. One told me to exercise more, another insisted that I take prescription medication, and one recommended thousands of dollars' worth of herbs. These were not the answers I expected. I was looking for a fresh and new approach—one based on my personal needs, not a generalized treatment plan.

I cannot even begin to articulate how this outcome made me feel. I said to myself, "This must be a joke. Has anyone done their due diligence to look over my medical history with a fine-tooth comb?" I started looking around to see if I could spot hidden cameras. I must be on *Candid Camera* or ABC's *What Would You Do?* This could not be real. It must be a test of my endurance or to see if I can withstand the constant blows. I asked myself, "Does anyone remotely know how badly I feel inside? Something is terribly wrong with me, and I must get to the bottom of this." Underlying sickness had gone on too long, and I felt it was beginning to permeate my entire body right under the watchful eyes of my team of experts.

Exasperated and Disheartened

The pain and disease were no longer isolated in certain parts of my body. They were expanding and becoming systemic. I knew it was impossible to diagnose myself. Trust me. If I could, I would. That's why I choose experts to help me in areas where I am not proficient. All I knew to do was to tell each specialist which symptoms I was having, and as new ones arose, I communicated those to them also.

Each doctor's visit left me exasperated and disheartened. My greatest joy was initially setting out to pursue specific doctors.

Reading the biographical sketch of each practitioner and what they claimed they could do for patients made my exploration new and exciting. My heart palpitated and leapt for joy as I read testimonials from past and current clients. My outlook became hopeful and promising. Searching for new doctors made me feel as if I was actively accomplishing a task that would ultimately lead to the answers I longed for.

Yet when it was all said and done, I was left deeply disappointed and bewildered. All the work and effort I put in appeared futile. When no one was able to help me, it seemed as if I was pushed back to square one. I often asked Lew, "How is it that all these other people are getting the help they need except for me? Others are seeing tremendous results, and I'm not."

"That's because no one is willing to go deeper with you," he said, "to take the time to dig further to find out what's really going on."

A Frightening Episode

I continued to make my yearly doctor's appointment, hoping that one day something magnificent would happen for me. I looked for ways to keep my spirits up, to keep the door of despondency tightly shut, because one crack in that door would literally drain the life out of me. Like biblical Abraham and Sarah, I hoped "against all hope" (Romans 4:18 NIV).

In between each doctor's visit, strange things continued to happen, which confirmed I was in full-blown tipping point status. One day at work, I felt a sharp pain in my left eye. (I once heard a comedian say that everything bad that happens to you happens on the side of your dominant hand. You probably have figured out by now that I'm left-handed.) The pain grew increasingly worse. Within seconds, I saw a long beam of light emanating from my eye to the point that it impaired my vision. The light was reminiscent of a heat wave I had seen as I looked outward on a hot summer day. With my eyes wide open, I felt around, looking for my desk so I could sit and gather my composure. This was, by far, the weirdest feeling I ever felt. With the blinding light, I also experienced what I can only describe as an electrical shock. I felt like I had gone into another dimension.

It took almost an hour to pass. Once I regained my full sight, I called Lew on his cell phone and frantically described to him what I had experienced. I said, "Something is terribly wrong with me.

"What?" The panic in Lew's voice was obvious.

"I have to get help immediately," I said. "I went blind in one eye, and now my sight is just starting to come back." I had never gone through anything like that, and I was not sure if it could occur again that day while I was still at work. Therefore, I informed him that should anything further happen to me my purse and other valuables were in the bottom drawer of my desk. "I'll leave the key on top of my desk so you can find it should you have to come and get me."

After we ended our call, I went downstairs to my principal's office and revealed to her what had happened. She escorted me to the nurse's office and told me I needed to be examined as a precaution. The school nurse checked my blood pressure and blood sugar. Both readings turned out normal. I went back upstairs to my office and contacted my eye doctor. I gave him a detailed rundown of what I had gone through. He insisted he wanted to see me right away.

Within two days, I had an emergency appointment with my ophthalmologist. I was afraid the spontaneous light would happen again and did not want to drive to the office alone, so I asked my cousin Belinda to drive me to my appointment. The ophthalmologist gave me a thorough eye exam. After the screening, he assured me everything appeared to be fine, and most importantly, my retina was still intact. Based on my symptoms, he called the event an "ophthalmic headache." Of course, he also advised, "Should it happen again, do not hesitate to call our offices." He also told me to go to a health food store and purchase lutein for my eyes. I always get excited when a doctor prescribes a supplement versus medication.

Before this crazy eye incident happened, most of my pain has been felt in my abdomen region, my left breast, and my lower back. With this sudden blindness, I could not help but think the worst. I told myself, "The pain has now migrated to my head area, which is currently affecting my eyes. Prior to this, my eyes have been fine. I didn't even need to wear corrective lenses. These doctors I have employed need to hurry up and figure out what's wrong with me. Whatever is ailing me is traveling upward."

Fortunately, the ophthalmic headache never returned. Migraines and lesser headaches persisted, but I refused to take any medications. As I mentioned before, my goal is not to avoid medications but to get to the root cause of the situation instead of masking it by numbing or removing the pain. I prefer to suffer through it and find a solution rather than to mistakenly think I'm getting better because I have lessened the pain.

A Different Kind of Blood Work

At my next primary care physician (PCP) appointment, when he asked how I was doing, I reported to him that I had gone blind in my left eye and that my eye doctor diagnosed it as an ophthalmic headache. "The headaches are nonstop," I said. "Overall, I still do not feel well. I have low energy, I'm not myself. I'm unable to lose weight, although I am careful about what I eat and exercise daily."

The doctor asked me to list everything I usually have for breakfast, lunch, and dinner. After I gave him a rundown of all three meals, he nodded as if to indicate his approval. One suggestion he made was to give up cold cereal and replace it with toast made from Ezekiel bread. He even had an empty sample bag to show me what to look for. He insisted it would be a better choice for me. I was willing to do whatever it took.

After he checked my vitals, he told his nurse the specific type of blood work he wanted drawn for me so she could prepare the right vials. The nurse drew my blood, put a bandage where the needle was inserted to be sure there was no further bleeding, and said they would call me with the results.

On my way home, I stopped by the supermarket and picked up the bread he had suggested along with a butter spread to be prepared for my morning meal. As I've done in times past, I patiently waited and hoped for the best. I always felt confident I was doing all I could do. The only thing left for me to do was wait for the results, then act accordingly.

Anything I commit to, I give it my all. I do not believe in cheating on myself. Once I set a goal, I stick with it wholeheartedly. This way of thinking has always been a part of my all-or-nothing nature. However, I became even more dogmatic because of the desperation that ran through my being as I sought answers for my health. One thing I won't do is indulge in cheat days. I find no value in them. I refuse to let my stomach and my desire ruin the outcome I long for. My satisfaction comes in knowing I have given it everything I possibly can. My faithfulness to the process gives me the confidence I need, knowing I have done all I can do. I always hold out the banner that maybe this time all the positive changes I've made will produce different results in my lab work and my overall well-being.

New Data Uncovered

Three weeks passed, and as promised, the doctor's office called with my results. Because I was at work, they left a message on my home answering machine to tell me I could either call them back for the results, or they could mail me a hard copy. I wanted both. When I spoke to the nurse, I was very disappointed when she informed me my blood work showed "everything looked normal except your LDL cholesterol was in a dangerous range and your liver enzymes were high, indicating that you have a compromised liver."

I had known about the cholesterol levels quite a while and had been working on bringing them down through diet and exercise, but the fact that they were at dangerous levels, even with a lifestyle change, was quite alarming. Having elevated liver enzymes left me perplexed. I asked myself, "How did I get elevated liver enzymes, and how do I rectify it?" I often associated liver disease with those who drink alcohol. My beverage of choice has always been plain water. I do not drink alcohol. Therefore, how did I get this unwelcome diagnosis? I later learned I was experiencing non-alcoholic fatty liver disease (NAFLD), which "is a buildup of extra fat in liver cells that is not caused by alcohol. It is normal for the liver to contain some fat. However, if more than 5%–10% of the liver's weight is fat, then it is called a fatty liver (steatosis)."[11]

Before we ended the call, the nurse also said the doctor wanted her to tell me my blood work indicated I had contracted the Epstein Barr Virus (mononucleosis).

"When?" I asked. "And how did that happen?"

"You got it when you were little, but right now it is dormant," the nurse responded.

According to the Center for Disease Control and Prevention (CDC), "diagnosing EBV infection can be challenging because the symptoms are similar to other illnesses. EBV infection can be confirmed with a blood test that detects antibodies. About nine out of ten adults have antibodies that show they have a current or past EBV infection."[12] I'm not sure what I said in the doctor's office to prompt him to test me for the antibodies to EBV, but I'm glad he did. The trigger to order that particular test may have been when I told him I have very low energy and I don't feel like myself. Throughout the years, I have had an extensive amount of blood work, but never did anyone test for EBV, so I had never been told I had been infected by this virus. I am so thankful he decided to test me for it.

Getting to the root causes of my medical issues has been a long and arduous process, but I refuse to give up. Every detail uncovered has proven to be a valuable tool to assist me in getting closer to the root cause. When I was growing up, mononucleosis was known in my school as a kissing disease, and since I never kissed anyone when I was younger, I thought it strange, first of all, that I even had it, and secondly, I was surprised the test showed it was contracted when I was younger. I jokingly told the nurse I must have caught it from one of my older sisters because we shared each other's food and drink.

In the days that followed, I continued to work on the areas that needed my attention as outlined by my blood work. In an effort to lower my LDL cholesterol, I increased my exercise to twice a day. I ran on my treadmill every morning for an hour before work. In the evening, Lew and I continued our three-mile walks, rain or shine. Although I was never a daily meat eater, I reduced my meat-eating to weekends only. I continued eating cheese and eggs freely because my doctor said neither had anything to do with my cholesterol levels being high. Lunch always consisted of a huge green salad and Greek yogurt for dessert. For dinner Monday through Friday, I added more variety. I ate peas and rice, beans and rice, pasta, vegetable chili, homemade pizza, roasted vegetables, sautéed kale, sweet potatoes, and other vegetable assortments. If I was still hungry after dinner, I ate fruit or a bag of microwave popcorn. Unfortunately, no one I had spoken with had any concrete answers on how to bring my liver enzymes down.

"Just a Blackhead"

I continued to modify my diet and stay on my exercise regime. When winter came, I noticed something was rubbing against the fastener on my bra. Like a contortionist, I reached my arm around my back to see if I could touch it to determine what it was. As the weeks progressed, this object on my back grew bigger. Finally, I asked Lew to take a look at it. He asked me to take my shirt and bra off and lean over the bathroom sink so he could get a good view of what was alarming me.

When he saw it, he shrugged off my concern by saying, "Oh, it's just a blackhead." He then insisted, "Stay where you are. I want to see something." He went to his side of the bathroom and opened his cabinet to tear off a piece of paper towel. He grabbed a cotton ball and some rubbing alcohol. He asked me to bend over further and lean on the sink so he could squeeze the lump on my back. When he did, I let out a bloodcurdling scream. I had never felt that kind of pain. He proudly showed me what he had extracted, and the look on his face said he was satisfied he had solved my problem.

The next day this so-called blackhead was back, but this time it was larger than the day before. Lew followed the same protocol. When he squeezed it this time, not only did I yell, but tears also flowed down my face. I said to him, "You know I have a high tolerance for pain. For me to cry like this, it must really hurt."

He agreed. He showed me the cotton ball. The content expelled was even greater. This time the whole cotton ball was filled with yellowish substance, which had a noticeable odor. Each day the lump on my back, near my spine, grew. I called my PCP to schedule an appointment for him to take a look at it and to refer me to a dermatologist. I wanted a real doctor to extract this blackhead, not "Dr. Lew."

A Sebaceous Cyst

When it was time for me to be examined, my doctor put on this weird device that looked like a set of goggles with magnifying glasses and lights. Whatever he was wearing on his face, it looked very official. I lay on the examining table face down. Before I could get situated to ask him a question, he blurted out, "Surgery tomorrow."

"What? For a blackhead!"

"That's not a blackhead," he said. "That's a sebaceous cyst, and it looks like someone has been messing with it."

I did not say a word. I was not going to throw "Dr. Lew" under the bus. When I got home, I told my husband that the thing he thought was a blackhead was a cyst, and I was going for surgery the next day.

He was in complete shock and disbelief. "Wow, I thought it was a blackhead because when I squeezed it, stuff came out," he retorted.

The next morning, I arrived for my appointment, and the nurse took me to a mini surgical room located toward the back of the doctor's office. I had no clue this makeshift operating room was on the premises. Notably, I was very calm. I was at peace and had no fear. The doctor assured me the hardest part was the huge needle he used to numb the area where he had to cut out the cyst. Surprisingly, I did not feel any pain. Once the numbing medication took effect, the doctor cut out the sebaceous cyst. When he had extracted it, he showed it to me and blurted out to the nurse, "To the lab stat."

What I saw was a dime-size purplish cyst that was perfectly round from Lew strategically trying to squeeze it out of my back.

The doctor closed the incision with a couple of stitches and bandaged the wound securely. He sent me home with explicit instructions on how to take care of the surgical area until it had completely healed.

The lab results came back quickly. Fortunately, the cyst was non-cancerous. That was the first good news I had received in quite some time. Although that news elated me, I still yearned to know what was going on in my body that caused all these out-of-the-ordinary things to happen to me in succession.

Chapter Five

Playing Whack-a-Mole

**I know for sure that in every challenging experience
there's an opportunity to grow, enhance your life,
or learn something invaluable about yourself.
Every challenge can make you stronger if you allow it.
Strength multiplied = power.[13]**

~ Oprah Winfrey

The time had come for my routine six-month dental checkup. This is one doctor my family and I look forward to seeing. Dr. Olivero and Colleen are like family to us. At the time of this writing, we have been with this practice for over twenty years. We love going together as a family. The three of us schedule our appointments on the same day back-to-back. The receptionist takes great care to find a date where she can fit us all in within half an hour apart. While one is in the chair, the other is usually visiting and talking until it's the other person's turn for cleaning. We absolutely love and trust our dentist.

Besides being the coolest dentist ever, Dr. Olivero along with his wife, Colleen, who is my dental hygienist, always take really good care of us. At the end of our cleaning, we often get a glowing report about how well we manage our dental home care. They consistently rave about how great we keep our teeth clean and how they can tell that we take our dental health seriously. Each visit, we laugh, joke, and catch up on what's happening that's new and exciting with each family member. Going to the dentist office is usually uncomfortable for most people, but I absolutely love it.

During this six-month routine exam, it was time for my yearly dental x-ray. While seated upright in the dental chair, my hygienist, Colleen, walked over to drape me with the large tan-colored weighted lead apron. As she covered the front of my body to shield my vital organs, I jokingly said, "Getting x-rays must be dangerous. First, you put this apron on me, and then you run out of the room before you capture the picture. What's up with that?" We got in a good chuckle as she continued taking x-rays of my upper and lower mouth. (After I was diagnosed with autoimmune disease, I stopped getting conventional x-rays, and I am going to a biological dentist who does digital x-rays until my dentist can go digital.)

A Spot on My Lower Gum

When all the x-rays were completed, Colleen came back into the room and lowered the chair to a reclining position in preparation for my cleaning. Shortly afterward, another hygienist came in with a set of x-rays and asked if they belonged to Colleen. As she looked over the film, it seemed as if there was a cosmic atmosphere shift in the room. You could hear a pin drop as she analyzed the skeletal-looking teeth of my x-ray.

She looked up for a second and then as she fixed her gaze back on the film, she penetrated the silence. "Hmm, something's showing up on your x-ray, but let's wait and let the dentist take a look at it."

With those words, I literally felt my heart skip a beat.

She called out to the corner office and asked the dentist if he had a moment to come into the room to take a look. He carefully looked over the x-ray and stated that in my lower gum the x-ray showed a spot. As I expected, based on his optimistic outlook, he went on to say, "It could be nothing. It could be a cyst."

Dr. Olivero knows all about my health history, and he and his wife are two of the most caring people I know. The hesitation on Colleen's part was because she knows how much I have gone through, and she did not want, in a million years, to be a bearer of bad news. I trust these professionals completely, so I'm always at ease when I'm in the dental chair.

Dr. Olivero continued, "Let's get it checked out first before we worry." He always has a positive and assuring attitude, and over the years he has shown a caring disposition toward me and my entire family. His understanding approach enabled me to trust him unwaveringly. A few moments later, he handed me my film and a referral to see a specialist. He smiled and said, "While you are waiting to get an appointment with the specialist, get yourself some sugar-free lemon drops and suck on those to see what happens."

"And you know I will," I remarked.

When I got home, I hurriedly pulled out my magnifying mirror and checked my lower gum frequently that day. I turned on every light in my bathroom, and I pulled my bottom lip as far out of the way as I could to be sure I got a clear view of my lower gum. Nothing abnormal stood out to me, but I saw the spot revealed on the x-ray. That night before bed, I took extra precaution when brushing my teeth. I did not brush my gum area too hard because I did not want to disturb what the x-ray had revealed. Neither did I want to cause the spot to get worse.

A Positive Prognosis

It wasn't long before I saw the specialist. He looked over the x-ray I had brought with me from the dentist, then he reclined my chair back as far as it would go and pulled the dental operatory light toward my mouth to get a closer look. I couldn't hear any outside noises because the loud sound of my heartbeat was deafening to my ears.

One of my life's missions has been to never let fear stop me. Although I repeatedly receive bad news from my doctors, I refuse to stop going. I continuously keep all of my appointments and yearly screenings. Healthwise, I've been through quite a lot. It seems that before I get a chance to recover from the news of one diagnosis, another different and worse diagnosis has been given. Repeated negativity with no breaks in between has caused fear to crop up. Fear will come. But it is up to me to not to let it petrify me. That's one of the ways I have been able to conquer my fear. I've put forth a lot of effort to not let it hold me back from moving forward. Nelson Mandela said, "I learned that courage was not the absence of fear, but the triumph over it. The brave man is not he who does not feel afraid, but he who conquers that fear."[14] I am determined to triumph over fear too.

The wait in the specialist's chair seemed like an eternity to me, but the examination of my gums was done within minutes. Just as my dentist had predicted, the specialist confirmed that what he saw on the x-ray was indeed a cyst, but his prognosis was more welcoming. He said the cyst should go away within a matter of time, and there was no need for him to perform gum surgery to remove it. He too recommended for me to incorporate lemon as part of my strategy for getting rid of it. He prescribed that I drink plenty of lemon water to flush the cyst out of my mouth.

I was elated beyond words. "Oh yes, sir, I definitely can and will do that," I muttered. With that wonderful news, I left his office with a special hallelujah on my lips and a song of praise emanating from my mouth. I was over-the-moon happy. Walking to my car to prepare to go home, I noticed that my head was held higher and my back was straighter than when I entered the medical offices. Outside, the sky seemed bluer and the white clouds fluffier. The birds sang so joyfully, and the afternoon sun's rays softly shined on my cheeks. It was indeed a perfect day to face the lion of fear and conquer it.

Another Meddlesome Attack

As foretold, in less than six months, the cyst in the lower region of my gums was totally gone. But to my dismay, another one had cropped up under my chin. I remember the day so vividly. School was about to start, and it was our extended family's custom to get together at my cousin's house to pray for the upcoming school year for our children. Since I was a teacher, the group included me in that prayer time. We fervently prayed for the safety of our children, we prayed that they would grow in their academics and character, and we prayed for their teachers that they would fully understand their subject matter and be able to teach each individual student according to the way each one learns. Lastly, we prayed that each of our children would give and receive respect from teachers and peers.

After our prayer time for the children ended, I asked for special prayer for me because I had found a hard pea-size lump under my chin. I asked them to pray that I stayed strong mentally and physically in the midst of all these attacks on my health. From what I had shared, I could clearly see the concern on my cousins' faces. In times past and to the present, they have been fully aware of all the fiery trials I have gone through with the different diagnoses. Now, this new discovery.

To them, all this bad news seemed like another meddlesome attack. Every time I shared a new diagnosis with them, they shook their heads in disbelief. They often said to me, "If I did not personally know you and your health concerns, there's no way that I could believe someone has gone through this much."

While we were in our circle of prayer, my cousin left her place in the circle and had the two children flanked on either side of her to join hands with each other while she came over to me to pray. As a point of contact, she put her hand under my chin and said, "Oh wow! I can feel the lump." When she prayed, she asked God to remove the lump and to totally heal me so I didn't have to continue to suffer.

Tears flowed profusely out of my eyes. I said out loud in the hearing of all who were present, "I am tired and don't know how much more I can take. I need a break from suffering."

The looks on everyone's faces and the shaking of their heads signaled they agreed with me that enough is enough.

That morning, I recalled the remedy my dentist and the specialist had me use for the cyst in my gums. Consequently, I chose the same treatment for the lump under my chin. This time, I upped the ante. Since lemon water worked so well in removing the cyst in my mouth, I had this epiphany that lemon juice is much more concentrated and should really get the job done.

Each morning, I ran several lemons through my cold press juicer until I extracted eight ounces. That may sound excessive, but I wanted to quickly remove that hard lump from under my chin. I was determined to drink this juice every day until I saw results.

Within approximately three weeks, the cyst was completely gone. The first people I called were my cousins Dion and Belinda to tell them that the cyst under my chin was gone and to thank them again for their prayers. With exuberant joy, I told the good news to as many as I could. All expressed how happy they were for me, but they could not help but pucker when I shared the method I had used.

In light of all the recurring cysts, I was reminded of the impromptu question I asked the surgeon who removed the cyst from my left breast: "Why do I keep getting cysts, and how do I prevent them?"

"Just Ignore Him"

The school year was well on its way, and it was time for me to go back to my PCP for another round of blood work. While there, I notified my doctor, hoping to motivate him to probe deeper since two more cysts had been found, one by my dentist and one by me. I told my PCP that one had appeared in my mouth, the other one under my chin. I also revealed that I daily drank eight ounces of lemon juice in an effort to flush out the cyst.

His negative reaction left me feeling that I should not have reported this to him. As an empath, I feel way more than what a person says. I pick up on people's energy, positive or negative. With this in mind, I had to put aside what I was sensing in order to divulge as much information as I could to get the medical help I so desperately needed.

He spoke to me about the results of my last labs and asked me what I was doing about it. I reiterated the ways I had changed my diet and continued my twice-daily exercise regimen. The more I talked, the more agitated he seemed to become. To everything I said, based on the question he asked, he responded with a sarcastic remark. Then he questioned and quizzed me on medical terms as if I had a degree in medical science. When I couldn't properly answer them, he seemed delighted.

To that end, the very thing that I was trying to reject began to physically overwhelm me. Under the circumstances, I gave him the benefit of the doubt and tried to stay positive, but I could not ignore what I felt in his presence. Ignoring the pop medical quizzes, I told him that my weight was not budging. Despite the fact that I had cut down on my food intake and portions, my stomach was getting bigger. "I always feel sick," I said. "I am weak with low energy, and my headaches are persistent."

He just stared at me.

In the quietness, I blurted out, "Is it my endocrine system? I think it's my endocrine system."

"No, you are fine. Your blood work says it's normal."

His retort made me feel very uneasy. "It's so strange that I'm having all these symptoms, and it's not being picked up in my blood work. The blood work is not even picking up all of these cysts," I said to myself.

He then sat down at his laptop and began to tap the keyboard.

I silently prayed, "Lord, please let him find the answer to my problems. It can't be me imagining these things because physical signs are confirming something is wrong. How can you ignore physical signs?"

Shortly after, he got up from his stool and left the room. This time he returned with the nurse. He listed, out loud, every blood test he wanted drawn. Then he left the room again.

This time I listened for footsteps to be sure he was out of earshot. When I felt it was safe to talk, I shared with the nurse the questions he had asked me and how he made me feel while he was quizzing me. "His harsh tone makes me feel bad, and I do not feel supported," I said.

"He must be having a bad day because he never acts like that," she replied.

Once all the vials of blood were filled, the nurse put a bandage on the spot where the needle was inserted to be sure that I did not bleed out. She said, "The doctor will contact you when the results are in."

I was not satisfied with the nurse's response to my comment about not feeling fully supported by my doctor, so when it was time to pay my copay, I shared the same sentiments with the receptionist.

"Oh, just ignore him," she said as she waved her hand.

"You Found a Good One, Babe"

In the meantime, I continued my search for doctors that I could add to my team and help me get to the root cause of all these strange, recurring happenings in my body. I went back to my computer and typed "Holistic Medical Doctors in My Area" in the Search box. As I scrolled through the list, one name caught my attention. Unfortunately, the practice was located in Virginia Beach, a two-hour drive from where I live.

When I checked the web page for office hours, I noticed the practice was closed on the weekends. Therefore, when I was ready to make the appointment, I would have to take a day off from work. I've traveled to Virginia Beach plenty of times, and I know that the traffic from the capital city to the Tidewater area can be grueling during the week due to bumper-to-bumper traffic, especially during business hours.

After reading the menu of patient services on the website, I was motivated to call and make an appointment despite the time it would take me to get there. What specifically caught my eye was the fact that the doctor's website declared that he holistically treats the whole person. He also highlighted specific areas of expertise he offered. The two that stood out to me were breast health and weight loss. After thoroughly reading the website's content and the doctor's biography, I called and made my appointment. The receptionist asked me to fill out the new patient information online so it would be in their office before I arrived.

Lew and I left before the crack of dawn to be sure I was on time for my 8:00 a.m. appointment. To pass the time, we talked and listened to our favorite music playlist. Although we did hit some traffic when we got on Interstate 64, we were not alarmed because we left early enough to compensate for traffic delays. In addition, we were so excited to find a doctor that treated the whole person that we did not care how far we had to travel. Lew and I were confident we were going to finally get answers to my health challenges, so he was willing to do just about anything. While driving to Virginia Beach, he said, "I'll drive you to New York if we can find a doctor that can help you."

We made it just in time for my appointment, with no time to spare. When we walked into the building, we were met with a warm welcome from the receptionist. When I walked up to her desk, she called me by my name. I knew then that I was in the right place, and that this medical practice pays attention to detail. She went on to reassuringly say, "We are glad that you are here. You are in good hands. The doctor is so thorough that he will peel back your layers of sickness like an onion."

Wow! Lew and I were delighted. That news was so refreshing. It was music to my ears. *I'm getting ready to get some help now.*

Once we said our hellos, she pointed to a nearby chair, told me to have a seat, and said, "The doctor will be with you shortly."

Lew and I kept eyeing each other and whispering, "Can you believe this? What a breath of fresh air!" He added, "I think you found a good one, babe."

Unbelievable Advice

A few minutes later, the doctor came out to the receptionist area, introduced himself, and took us into his office. With my medical records in hand, the doctor sat with me and read over each report. As he combed through each record, he looked up occasionally to ask a question about anything that stood out to him.

We were literally there for hours.

Prior to this, no medical doctor had ever taken that much time to go over my records, especially with me present. Once he finished going over the first stack, he kept flipping the last page over as if he wanted more to appear. Finally he said, "Is that it?"

"Well, yes, that's a huge file. What else should I have brought?"

"All the testing is the same," he explained. "Did your PCP do any other testing?"

"No, he didn't. I only have what's in my file."

He asked me a series of pertinent questions about my symptoms and then proceeded to write up specific tests he needed to make a fair and accurate assessment. He didn't accept any insurance, but he did not want me to bear the burden of any out-of-pocket expenses. So, to save me money from paying for my blood tests, he asked me to go back to my PCP and have him draw the specific labs he wanted so he could further analyze what was going on in my body without extra out-of-pocket expenses for me.

When we got up to leave, we shook hands. He walked us back to the receptionist area where we made my next appointment to go over the new blood work he wanted my PCP to order.

At the end of our meeting, I was exhausted. The long ride and the many questions from the doctor were taking their toll on me. I felt excruciating pain in my entire body, and we had another two-hour return trip ahead of us. Our time frame for the trip back home was totally dependent on the amount of traffic. As we contemplated the long ride home, I recalled the last and most exhilarating recommendation the doctor left me with. He said, "Stop exercising so much."

When we got back to the car, I called my sister Beverly in Florida. She was at work, so I knew I had to make this call very brief. On the third ring, she picked up the phone. She hardly had a chance to say hello before I jumped in and said, "Girl, guess what? I found another doctor for my team, and you won't believe the recommendation he gave me."

My sister started laughing and giggling as she tried to figure out what he could have told me, but she was taking too long to figure it out. I couldn't take it anymore. I finally gave it away. "He told me to stop exercising so much. Can you believe that?"

"What medical doctor is going to tell a patient to stop exercising so much?" I repeatedly asked.

My sister assured me, "For him to say that, there must be something to it."

Years later, I found out that my sister was absolutely right. There was something to what that doctor said about exercising too much. When you have thyroid disease and low adrenals, too much exercise can be detrimental instead of beneficial.

Devastating News

In the days ahead, I received a phone call from my PCP that the blood work results he had ordered were in and he was ready to go over them with me. This was perfect timing because I could use this visit to share with him the good news that I had added another doctor to my team and he wanted my PCP to order labs for him. What perfect timing!

During my appointment, my PCP said, "Your labs show that your LDL cholesterol is still climbing." This time, my doctor was adamant that I should be on medication. He said, "You've worked long enough on your own to fix it, and since dietary changes and exercise have not worked, medication is now the way to go."

This seemed like a perfect time to inform him that I had added a new doctor on my team and he wanted to order these labs. As I handed him the order form, he said, "If he wants these tests, have him order them himself." He then returned the lab order sheet to me.

Needless to say, I was devastated. I had high hopes that this new doctor was going to get to the bottom of everything I was experiencing. *If I do not get these labs, what am I going to do?* I had no idea I would be met with this impasse. I didn't have the extra money to pay for more labs. After all, that's why I pay for insurance to cover the tests I need.

I could not convince my PCP to change his mind, so I moved on and asked him if he could give me three more months to continue working on my health to see if there was any improvement before I even talked about the prospect of taking medication.

As I've said in previous chapters, I am by no means opposed to medication, but I know that before anything is prescribed, the root cause should be discovered. Why is my cholesterol climbing on a healthy diet that also includes exercising?

My PCP unwaveringly refused to order the labs requested by another doctor, and I left his office feeling so defeated. I felt like my world had just crashed down on me and the universe was against me getting the help I needed.

I knew that seeking additional help was not wrong. "It's my body," I told myself, "and I can see anyone who is willing to give me the help I need. I am not tied to one physician. I'm trying to build a team of experts. I need help, and time is of the essence."

A Letter Written But Never Sent

That afternoon, I sat down at my computer and composed a two-page letter to my PCP asking him why he would refuse help to someone who is desperately seeking it. Why would he not order those labs for me? In the letter, I shared how I was strategically gathering a team of doctors to help me with the health challenges I had battled since the tender age of thirteen and longer. I enumerated how each blood work, test, and screening indicated that I was getting progressively worse. I went on to say, "I thought your medical goal was to help me find a solution to what has been causing these imbalances in my body. If that is indeed your goal, then why would you deny me any resources to help meet that mutual goal?" While typing the letter, I felt empowered and justified. My goal was to help him see that my objective and concern were to get the answers to this overwhelming health challenge, not to hurt him in any way.

Actually, it wasn't about him. It was about me and my health. I wanted him to understand that each diagnosis was a blow to me emotionally and physically and having further diagnostic testing would give me the clarity I needed, especially from a medical doctor who was willing to probe further.

After the letter was completed, I went into the kitchen to get the cordless phone to call the doctor's office to ask the receptionist for the mailing address so I could send it right away. When the receptionist, who is the main reason I remained as long as I did in this practice, answered the phone, I told her about the letter and the reason I was writing it. Before she gave me the address, I asked if I could read it to her before sending it. She agreed.

When I finished reading it, she encouraged me not to send it. Although I so desperately wanted to send it because it allowed me to say how important it is for a doctor to listen to his patients and to list in detail all I had experienced, I acquiesced because I trusted her. She has always been professional, kind, and courteous toward me. For example, if the doctor recommended a specialist, she made sure it was one that fit my needs and personality.

I respected her request, but I also wanted to send the letter because I wanted a voice. I wanted to educate the doctor as to the importance of working together with other professionals to achieve the health goals of the patient. I also wanted to send the letter because I felt that all the diagnoses were dictating what I was going to do or what was going to be done to me, but I did not have a voice of my own. I was being manipulated by sickness and disease. I did not understand her reason for saying, "Do not send it," but I trusted her. Her calls were always prompt and timely. Again, she was one of the primary reasons I stayed as long as I did in that practice, especially since year after year I saw no favorable medical results.

The next day, I called the doctor's office in Virginia Beach and told the receptionist to cancel my upcoming appointment because there was no need for me to come if additional tests were needed to evaluate me, and I was not able to get them from my PCP. The receptionist was baffled by the doctor's unwillingness to accommodate me by getting the labs I needed.

A Dangerously Low Heart Rate

More unusual occurrences continued to happen to me. Frustration set in because I was not able to get the help I needed. With each passing day, I felt like I was playing Whack-a Mole. Every time I was diagnosed with one health problem, another one seemed to pop up.

One day after work had ended, I was in the library getting ready to go home. Two teachers came up to talk to me about collaborating on a class project. As one was talking, the entire room went black. When I opened my eyes, I found myself on the scantily padded concrete floor face up with the other teachers staring at me. For a moment, I vaguely heard one of them calling my name. Once I became fully conscious, out of sheer embarrassment, I quickly jumped up and left the teachers standing there shaking their heads. They were perplexed as to what had happened. I walked into my office and found some almonds left over from my lunch in my bag and ate them. When I turned around, the two teachers were standing in my office, ready to finish sharing their collaboration ideas with me.

I was not alarmed about fainting because it had happened so quickly, and once I regained consciousness, it did not seem as if anything was wrong. I assumed that I had fainted due to hunger. While the teachers remained in my office, I called my PCP to let him know I had just fainted and asked him, "What do you think I should do?"

Since I called around 3:30 p.m., I was given an appointment that same day. Without any thought, I drove myself to the doctor's office. When I arrived, the waiting room was empty. The receptionist had already signed me in, and I was taken to the examination room right away. The doctor rolled in with the EKG machine, took my vitals, and hooked me up to the EKG machine. While the results were being read, he asked me to go over with him exactly what happened. I said, "Two teachers came up to talk to me, and while one was talking, I fainted. When I woke up, everyone in the room was staring at me."

When the EKG was done, my doctor tore off the perforated sheets of paper with the readings and gave it to me along with a referral to a cardiologist. He sent me to this specialist because my heart rate was alarmingly low. That explained why I had fainted.

Encouraging Results But No Root Cause

I waited until the next day to call the cardiologist because by the time I got home, their offices were closed. To my delight, the doctor was able to see me right away. I had never been to a cardiologist; therefore, I did not know what to expect. The waiting room was filled with a lot of elderly people, so I felt out of place. Many of the ones waiting to be seen appeared to also have a caregiver who assisted them in walking.

My wait to see the doctor was extremely long. Finally, after hours of waiting, the nurse called my name to escort me into the examination room. After she took my vitals and asked a few questions, the door opened and in walked the nicest, most apologetic doctor I've ever met. He apologized profusely for having me wait so long. I assured him that it was okay. He asked me quite a few probing questions, so his thorough intake was well worth the wait.

The moment I met him, I could tell he cared deeply for each patient. He exemplified his concern for the whole person—spirit, mind, and body. He continued to ask questions to try to get to the bottom of why I had fainted. When he finished his questioning, he told me that he would have to monitor my heart to see if he could detect any changes that were out of the ordinary.

Before I left his office, I was outfitted with a twenty-four-hour Holter heart monitor with wiring everywhere and several electrodes taped to my chest. Wow! I had never seen anything like that. It was like something right out of science fiction.

The next day I had to wear it to work, and when my students saw all the electrodes and wires, they were greatly concerned. I assured them it was not as scary as it looked. The doctor told me I had to wear the monitor for twenty-four hours, but I could do everything I normally did, so I should continue with my activities as usual. The only thing I couldn't do was get the equipment wet.

On the first day I wore the monitor, Mikayla and I went for our usual three-mile walk after school. Despite no clouds in sight and a favorable weather forecast, it unexpectedly started to rain. I was fully aware that the doctor said, "Do not get the monitor wet," and while walking, I kept repeating that directive to Mikayla.

Our three-mile walk turned into a three-mile sprint. The rain turned into a torrential downpour. For extra protection from the rain, Mikayla took off her jacket so I could cover up the monitor to keep it dry. We ran back home as fast as we could. Thankfully, we made it safely before the deluge descended on us with such ferocity that not even the extra jacket could protect the equipment.

I returned the monitor to the cardiologist's office the next day. When the nurse took it from me, she said, "The doctor will read the results and then be in touch with you." The following afternoon, I received a phone call from the doctor, and he gave me a detailed account of his findings. In the middle of the assessment, he paused and said, "May I ask you what you were doing between four and five o'clock yesterday?"

I facetiously replied, "Doctor, I cannot share that with you. That's my private business."

He said, "The reason I'm asking is because the monitor spiked really high during that time frame."

I let out a heartfelt laugh and said, "My daughter and I went for our three-mile walk and were caught in the rain. I recall you having one stipulation—'Don't get the monitor wet.' Well, we ran all the way home from our three-mile walk."

The doctor and I laughed hysterically.

Before we hung up the phone, he said, "Your heart is fine, and I do not usually say this to my patients, but you do not have any need to return to my office." He also said he would send over his findings to my primary care physician.

Once again, my body seemed to be sending overt messages that something was wrong, but no one had yet been able to get to the root cause of why all my systems from head to toe were on full alert.

When medical science has no answer for me, where do I go for help? Fatigue, low energy, cysts, high cholesterol, liver disease, weight gain—I always felt like I was dying, yet I had to drag my body through a world that moved on without me. According to Barbara Kingsolver, "The very least you can do in your life is figure out what you hope for. And the most you can do is live inside that hope. Not admire it from a distance but live right in it, under its roof."[15]

I hoped for health but the distance between wanting it and obtaining it seemed light years away.

Chapter Six

Divine Intervention

The first step in solving a problem is to recognize that it does exist.[16]

~Zig Ziglar

The constant health challenges and the quest to find answers were cause for fear and anxiety. Not having a medical diagnosis that corroborated the symptoms I was experiencing led to a lot of frustration and angst. Days on end, I sat and shook my head in disgust because it seemed as if my options were running out. I did not know what else to do. I was still experiencing meteor showers of pain. History kept repeating itself.

At the age of thirteen, I became aware of my body and how it was supposed to function. I did not fully understand it, but the first indisputable indication that something was amiss was when my menstrual cycle showed signs of irregularity. I instinctively knew my body was not functioning optimally like the bodies of others around me. The girls my age had their menstruation come like clockwork, month by month. They knew the exact day it would show up. That information was not afforded to me. Mine was sporadic, and at times, it would not come at all for months.

I remember telling my mom, "My menstrual did not come this month." She did not even flinch. It appeared she was not alarmed by this. Each time my period was absent, I brought it to my mom's attention. Again, no response. After repeated times of no acknowledgment or concern from my mom, I decided it was useless to keep repeating something that seemed to have no impact on her. So, I stopped telling her. She never even inquired if it ever came or not.

I eventually moved on from her and shared the news sporadically with my sisters. They too seemed unmoved. One sister did tell me not to worry about my menstruation not coming. But how could I not be distressed by its absence?

I innately knew that having an irregular menstrual cycle was not normal or healthy. Plus, its infrequency was coupled with bouts of feeling sick. I was so happy when it did come that I heralded to everyone, "My period came, my period came."

Those that had a regular menstrual cycle did not welcome it like I did. I was elated and excited mainly because I felt my body was doing what it was programmed to do. I equated having a monthly cycle with being healthy because afterward I always felt better than I did before it came. After it came and went, I sensed an inner cleanliness. Having my monthly period made me proud to be a girl. During and after, I felt like a grown woman.

There were unpleasant times also, but I never let those times get the best of me. Unfortunately, my menstrual cycle was accompanied by hard stomach cramping and huge blood clots that looked like liver. Oftentimes, I was forced to stay in bed, balled up in a fetal position as I tried to rock the pain away. Nonetheless, I still welcomed it. The positive side effects far outweighed the negative ones. I was so happy to have it finally come that I was willing to take the good and the bad. Like a long-lost friend, I was glad to see it.

On the other hand, I never witnessed anyone double over in pain as I did during the onset of my menstrual cycle. I had to find out why I was so different. Being the junior investigative reporter that I was, I interviewed family and friends to inquire if they too had cramps and blood clots. Some said they had mild cramps on the first day of their menses, while others did not. All of them unanimously agreed that they did not experience blood clots at all. I continued to bring up the subject of my menstrual cycle. I consistently divulged to one family member or another, "I'm not experiencing a regular menstrual cycle." Still, I was given no reaction or remedy from them.

The Seventh Basic Need

The continuation of other people ignoring my symptoms marked the beginning of a pernicious pattern that was repeated from childhood to adulthood. This is one of the main reasons I do not trust easily. In the most crucial times of my life, I never felt heard. When I needed dire help, it was not available to me. Everyone else seemed to live out their lives ignoring the harsh reality that something was seriously wrong with me. This signified for me the first fruit of a cycle of not being fully heard and acknowledged concerning my health. The grassroots started with my family and spread like weeds into my dealings with the medical profession.

According to psychologist Abraham Maslow, "Being heard" does not fall into the category of Maslow's Hierarchy of Needs: physiological (food and clothing), safety (employment, security), love and belonging needs (friendship), esteem, and self-actualization."[17] But I must take the liberty to add "being heard" to his list as a seventh basic need. When one is acknowledged and heard, it brings a high level of security. When I am fully heard, it makes me feel calm inside. Knowing that the person I'm sharing personal information with is not fully present leaves me nervous and jittery. Conversely, when I am heard, I experience calmness and validity. This allows me to flourish inwardly on a whole different level.

Years of experience have taught me that the chronological age of the person sharing the pertinent information has no bearing on whether that person should be "heard" or not. My health challenges started at a very young age and went undetected for years. One of the major reasons I assembled a medical team was in the hopes of finally being heard about my uncharacteristic symptoms that began to develop back in the 1970s.

These symptoms were serious and needed urgent attention. When a patient describes symptoms he or she is experiencing, medical protocol should never outweigh the action needed to get to the root cause and to take appropriate actions to alleviate the symptoms. Every time I had to repeatedly explain my symptoms yet received no response, I experienced undue stress, emotionally and physically. I felt like I was on a hamster wheel with no way to get off.

Happily, for decades, I did not succumb to the systemic physical pain. I did my best to not let the pain get the best of me. I did everything a person that was pain free would do, and I did it with a smile. Tolerating pain and discouragement have been a way of life for me. However, that is not ultimate living; it is a low-voltage ability to show a high level of endurance. When sharing my story with others, I stated the facts, but I never complained.

After years of not being heard coupled with the intense, increasing physical pain, my tolerance level began to wane. The physical pain coupled with not getting help for my physical condition started to break me down emotionally. This "tell me what you are going through, but I'm not going to do anything about it" mentality left me emotionally bankrupt. I faithfully kept my three-month, six-month, and yearly checkups, and I divulged all my symptoms and pain but received no corresponding action. This eventually had a negative impact on me. I became very concerned that the delay in getting help would push me to a place of no return because the help I needed was not afforded to me. I was petrified with the fear that I would one day go to a doctor's office and list all my symptoms, only to hear that medical professional say, "We have a diagnosis, but the disease has progressed beyond being treated." I could not bear to hear someone say, "It's too late."

I do not like being involved in anything that doesn't produce results, so I was always left asking, "What's the point?" This mindset stemmed from my success-oriented personality. Everything I do must be productive and fruitful. I like to see results in all my efforts. If I do not see the outcome I'm working toward, I am distressed, especially when I detect that my invested time and energy have been wasted.

Shabbat Shabbos

Early one morning following a good night's sleep, Lew and I woke up before our alarm clock chimed. Our eyes simultaneously popped open. Turning our heads toward each other, we silently acknowledged that we were fully awake and were not going back to sleep. My husband sprang out of bed to do his ritual morning prayer.

Spontaneously, without thought, I jumped up to join him. The room was dark, yet light from the large lamppost on our neighbor's front lawn was faintly shining through our closed blinds, enabling us to see objects in our room. It also projected just enough light to allow us to visually find our way around the room without bumping into furniture or stubbing our toes.

Lew and I love to walk and pray. Therefore, that shimmer of light was all we needed to enable us to see so we would not bump into each other in passing. Praying while walking empowers us. The movement makes us feel as if we are making great strides and accomplishing exactly what we set out to do. Walking while praying in the wee hours of the morning also keeps us laser focused and prevents us from drifting back to sleep.

While we were praying, I intermittently opened my eyes to be sure I was not moving too close to Lew. I wanted to stay within the small space I had allotted for myself. When I looked up, I noted that Lew was at a safe distance on the opposite side of the room. I'm not sure how long we were engaged in prayer, but it must have been some time because I was beginning to get tired from walking.

With my eyes still shut, I was able to safely walk over to my side of the room so I could continue praying while leaning on my dresser. As I reached out my hand to locate the corner of my dresser, something inexplicable happened. My subdued early morning prayer unexpectedly turned into a grievous wail and a heart-rending cry. My mouth was saying one thing, but my heart was screaming, "Lord I need your help. I am tired of going to all of these doctors, and no one is giving me the help that I need. I have spent so much money and time to no avail. You are my Creator. Help me, or I won't be able to continue like this."

Within seconds, I was enraptured. I could no longer feel the wood of my dresser underneath my hand. My body seemed to be suspended between heaven and earth. Beyond a shadow of doubt, the Divine had responded to my heartfelt cry. I unequivocally knew that the lifelong desire to "be heard" was met this day, not by a human being but by the Creator of the Universe.

There was a notable cosmic shift in our room. The atoms seemed to bow to the very presence of their Creator. Like the apostle Paul in the New Testament of the Bible, I was not sure if I was on earth or in heaven (see 2 Corinthians 12:3). Our family prayer time turned into an encounter. I did not want it to end. The awe and wonder I experienced were breathtaking.

For a split second, I glanced up to locate Lew. He was in a trance, unable to move. He could not utter a word, yet his affirming look indicated to me that indeed something was happening that was way bigger than us. Spirit to spirit we communicated that something supernatural was happening.

I turned my face back toward the wall behind my dresser, still crying and muttering distinct words that I had never before heard or spoken. Over and over, I kept saying the words, "*Shabbat Shabbos.*" I repeated those words innumerable times.

At that time, my finite mind thought it quite unusual that I kept saying those words so much. To this day, I believe that the purpose of the repetition was to etch the words indelibly on my heart and mind long after the prayer had ended. I had to say them multiple times because they were unfamiliar to me in their combined form, and repetition was the only way I could remember them.

The intense crying, praying, and walking expended a lot of energy, but somehow Lew and I felt refreshed and joyful afterward. When our prayers ceased and the aura in our room lifted, we staggered from our corners of the room and met in the middle to enjoy a long embrace.

"Wow! God met us here!" he said.

We glowed in the light of what had just transpired. As we held each other, we talked about the unfamiliar words that proceeded from my mouth, and we shared how we longed to know their meaning and intent for our lives. We wished it was the weekend so we could have remained and talked for hours.

Cognizant of the passing time, we quickly took our showers and got ready to go to work. As we rushed out the door to get into our respective cars, we whispered the words, "*Shabbat Shabbos,*" while saying our goodbyes with pointed fingers.

Exuberantly Happy

Those words stayed with me all day. At work, I found myself reliving and rehearsing what had happened early that morning. The joy I experienced was inexpressible. I felt like I had been kissed by heaven. I desperately wanted to know what the words meant to us and for us. Having traveled to Israel, I knew the word *Shabbat* in Hebrew meant "rest," but I had no idea what *Shabbos* meant.

That evening before dinner, I scoured the internet to find the meaning of *Shabbos*, and I kept coming up with no viable hits. Finally, I found a couple of websites that told me the meaning. In one of the articles, I read that *Shabbos* is the Yiddish word for the Hebrew Sabbath.[18]

Later I found an elaborate explanation of the word *Shabbos* that closely reflected the cry of my heart during my encounter when the words "*Shabbat Shabbos*" were divinely proceeding out of my mouth. "Shabbos ... represents an endpoint. ... It is not simply rest, inactivity. It is the celebration of the work which has been completed. ... A process must have an endpoint to give it meaning. If work never achieves a result, the work is foolish. ... So Shabbos teaches that all work must be directed to a goal."[19]

During our glorious early morning prayer time, my greatest request was to get a reprieve from the intense work I had been doing for my health and to be heard by my medical team regarding the symptoms I was experiencing so they could get to the root cause. Learning the meaning of those Hebrew words caused me to be exuberantly happy. What are the chances of these particular unfamiliar words being placed in my mouth to echo the desire for rest I had longed for since the age of thirteen?

Those words coupled with the encounter have had a lasting and sustainable effect on me. Prayer is an aperture to the lens of my spiritual eyes to see beyond what this world has to offer. It is the Messiah alone who has changed the topography of my life-torn heart. That unusual encounter gave me the will and the strength to carry on despite my past and whatever lay ahead.

The Most Troubling Phone Call

One Friday while at work, I got the most troubling call from Lew. He told me my niece had called and informed him that my mother had been rushed to the hospital. I couldn't believe what I was hearing. The utterance of those words made it seem as if the ceiling was falling in on me. *This can't be happening. I've never even seen my mother sick. How can she be in the hospital?*

"Are you sure?" I asked. "She must have the wrong mother. Not my mother!" I whimpered.

"We need to get to South Carolina ASAP," he said. "Leave work now. I'll pick up Mikayla, and you meet us at home so we can pack our clothes and go."

I hung up the phone and stood in my office engulfed in a cloud of disbelief. I was rehearsing and replaying every word Lew had said. "Mom has been rushed to the hospital." The sound of students talking outside my office brought me back to reality. My stomach started to spasm. My mouth became dry, my persistent headache intensified, and the room began to spin. My world seemed to crumble. Dazed by the sudden news, I unthinkingly left my office, passed the circulation desk, walked down the stairs and out the front door of the building, then drove home.

With a one-track mind and overcome by deep sadness, I forgot to notify the main office of the news I received. Neither did I tell them I was leaving. While we packed, Lew asked me, "What did the assistant principal say when you told him what happened?"

"Oh no, I didn't even tell him that I was leaving." I immediately called the school to apologize for walking out without first letting somebody know where I was and to say I was remiss in following protocol to sign out when leaving the building. The secretary answered the phone, and I explained to her all that transpired. I went on to say that my mother had been rushed to the hospital and that I was headed out of town to be by her side until she recovered.

When we left Virginia and headed south, the skies were gray and gloomy, yet the air was dry. As soon as we passed South of the Border and crossed the state line, the heavens opened and rain fell fast and furious, like a monsoon. It seemed as if the earth was crying for my mother. The rain beat vehemently upon our car from the time we arrived in South Carolina until we reached our destination.

"She's Not Responding"

Lew drove the entire trip with zero visibility. I offered to give him a break by taking my turn to drive. He refused because he wanted me to relax the best I could under the circumstances. He also wanted me to be available to tend to the needs of Mikayla, who quietly sat in the back seat soaking in everything that was going on. When we were halfway there, we received a call from my aunt who said, "They moved your mother to a hospital in Charleston that is better equipped to treat her condition. Dawn, she's not responding. It does not look good."

I begged her not to talk like that. "We must stay positive," I yelled.

With my mom being transported to Charleston, we had to drive another two hours to reach her. The sad news about my mom made the car ride very dismal. As I sat in the front seat, I became increasingly jittery and nervous. The seat belt harnessed from my shoulder to my waist did not prevent me from constantly rising up out of my seat to change positions. I was restless. I just couldn't keep still.

Arriving by plane would have gotten us there much sooner, but with such short notice, to get there without delay, we were forced to drive. With the anticipation of seeing my mom, it seemed as if we would never get there. It felt as if the car was moving in reverse, although we were driving the 65-mph speed limit when the rain permitted.

My reflexes were on full throttle. I kept pressing my right foot to the floor of my imaginary accelerator as if I were driving. I felt an urgency to see my mother, and it was not happening quickly enough. Maintaining a safe driving speed was paramount because the deluge was slowing us down due to limited visibility. The windshield wipers, although set on fast speed, could not keep up with the amount of water falling onto our car. I felt as if we were racing against time. It seemed as if even the darkness was getting darker.

Anxiety was getting the best of me. My heart felt like it was pounding out of my chest and about to burst. My breathing was increasingly heavier. I could not stop sighing. The pressure was becoming unbearable. *I'm hyperventilating. I have to see my mother right now. It's urgent. Come on, let's go. Hurry up.* These words played on repeat in my mind for the remainder of the trip.

Every so often Lew took his attention off the road to glance at me, checking to see if I was okay. He reached out to hold my hand in an effort to comfort me.

"Hold on, Mommy," I said out loud. "I'm coming. I'll be there shortly. Please hold on."

We arrived at the hospital at midnight. I was thankful and relieved we arrived safely on such a dangerous rain-soaked trip. The entire Lowcountry was flooded, making it difficult to find a parking spot where you did not have to get out of the car in ankle-high waters. We kept circling around trying to find parking. Finally, through the downpour, we saw signs that read Hospital Parking Garage.

"Mommy, I'm Here"

We own a minivan, so we usually aim for the biggest spot that gives us room to maneuver. That night we parked the minivan in the first available space we spotted. Lew helped our daughter from the back seat, and leaving everything else behind, we ran as fast as we could to the hospital entrance.

When we got off the elevator, we rushed toward the intensive care unit. The greeting from the nurses indicated they were eagerly awaiting our arrival. My mother was lying in the hospital bed, her room front and center of the nurses' station. From a distance, I saw all the machines she was hooked up to and the long breathing tube in her mouth.

I gently walked into her room and quietly exclaimed, "Mommy, I'm here!"

She slowly opened her eyes and looked intently at me. The words of my aunt—"she is unresponsive"—played back in my ears, but my eyes saw her respond to my voice. I was ecstatic. Bursting with excitement, I twirled around and danced for joy to physically see a bad report turn to good.

When I turned back around to continue to talk to my mom, her eyes were once again closed. For seven days, she never opened them again. During that heart-wrenching week, while she remained on life support, I couldn't sleep or eat. My health took a nosedive due to a lack of nourishment and no substantial rest. All my organs were physically stressed.

Watching my mom lie there with no movement day in and day out took a notable toll on me. We waited for the rest of my family to arrive from various parts of the country so decisions could be made collectively. It was difficult to see this vibrant woman, who worked up until this incident, lie there unresponsive. My mom was my best friend. As I got older, she had increasingly become my prayer partner and confidante.

A Collective Decision

Each day, the doctors' reports were increasingly bleak. "There's nothing else we can do," they said. My two sisters and my niece work in the medical field so they understood precisely what my mom's chart was projecting. After careful evaluations and brain scans, the doctors informed us that her brain bleed was getting progressively worse and should she remain on life support, her brain could rupture. We therefore made a collective decision to remove my mom from life support.

We had to support her wishes and stop any further suffering. Her life wasn't supposed to end like this. This was too tragic and unexpected. How would I go on without her? But to prolong her life like this was out of the question.

The day to remove her from life support was grueling and will forever and always be etched in my memory. We had back-to-back meetings from morning until late afternoon with the palliative care team in the hospital conference room. They thoroughly went over her condition and gave us a detailed account of what it was like when she arrived and how her health had declined. They projected on a huge screen her latest brain scans and other test results so we could clearly understand what they were describing. They went on to assure us that she would be heavily sedated before she was taken off life support so she would not experience any pain.

While they spoke, I wept. I was inconsolable. This was too final. My understanding of the medical jargon was impaired by my sadness. At times, I could hardly comprehend what the doctors said. I was preoccupied with the fact that I would never hear my mother's reassuring voice again. As the meeting came to an end, the doctors told us they would come and get us once they removed her from the life support so we could say our final goodbyes.

When I walked back into my mom's hospital room, I was able to see her full face because the tubing had been removed. When I thoroughly examined her lifeless body, hoping for a sign of life to appear, unprecedented fear gripped me. I felt bone-chilling cold in my extremities and throughout my entire body. The unexpected loss I felt was unspeakable. My siblings and I gathered around her hospital bed, Lew holding one of her hands and me holding the other.

It was our mission in her final moments to set a tone in her room she would have approved of, so we quietly sang her favorite songs and prayed for the angels to safely take her to the other side. Like a well-orchestrated symphony, each of us took turns reassuring her that it was okay to leave. We said, "This is the moment you have lived for. You will now get an opportunity to see your Lord and Savior." In less than an hour, flanked by her children, she slowly turned her head from one side to the other and breathed her last breath on earth and took her first breath in eternity. A week later, we laid her in her final resting place in her hometown where she was born.

A Psychiatric Referral

Following the homegoing services for my mom, I noticed I was starting to feel worse than ever. Through it all, I still kept repeating the words, *"Shabbat Shabbos."* Those words had become my mantra. They gave me such hope, and I held on to them for dear life.

I was unable to sleep at night, I was having unusual heart palpitations, and bouts of anxiety were taking over my life. I continually told Lew that my health was declining, although the medical testing was not picking up what I was describing. I said to him, "I look forward to *Shabbat Shabbos*. I desperately need the rest." He concurred.

One spring while I was teaching my class, I heard a muffled popping sound on the left side of the top of my brain. It seemed as if my blood vessels were stuck together and were trying to pull apart. I grabbed the top of my head, hoping the pressure from my hand would keep the blood vessels from bursting. I quickly walked to my office for fear that I was going to pass out in front of my students. I tried to be as inconspicuous as I could because I did not want to draw attention to myself.

With my hand now by my side, I peeked my head out of my office and told my students, "Keep working on your projects. I'll be right back." I closed my door and placed my hand on the spot where I heard the popping sound and prayed, "Lord, please heal me. Do not let me die at all, but especially at work."

Throughout the remainder of the day, I kept trying to take deep breaths to calm my body and mind. Fear gripped me and flashbacks of my mom lying in that hospital bed kept haunting me. My mom's cause of death was an aneurysm followed by a stroke. I shared this experience with no one because I did not want to give voice to it.

Later, I went for a checkup and shared with my doctor that my new symptoms were heart palpitations and anxiety attacks. I did not share the muffled popping sound in my head because I was too vulnerable to trust anyone with that information. I also divulged to him, "I'm always nervous, and my hands and feet are often cold." I repeated that my headaches were nonstop and I could not lose weight. The last thing I shared was that my hair was starting to fall out. "Do you think it's my thyroid?" I asked.

"No, the test says your thyroid is fine. I've tested it several times. You are fine."

With the rush of emotions, the passing of my mom, and the unexplained symptoms, I started crying uncontrollably.

"You need to go see a psychiatrist," he said as he walked out of the room, leaving me there bawling my eyeballs out.

How did my physical sickness now turn into a psychological one? I'm crying because no one is listening to me concerning the enormous number of physical symptoms I'm having.

Wait a minute!

Everything had happened so quickly. Left alone in the room, I looked around and said, "What just happened?"

The doctor came back in the room and said, "Your referral will be at the front desk."

A Difficult But Necessary Choice

That upcoming week was spring break, and I was looking forward to being with my family and hopefully catching up on some much-needed rest. After spring break ended, I was too sick to return to work. With no other recourse, I decided to go see the psychiatrist that was recommended.

My primary purpose for going was to be able to share once again all the symptoms I was experiencing with the hopes that after she evaluated me she would recommend the further testing I needed. She listened intently to everything I was dealing with both emotionally at work and in my physical health. She looked over my medical records and asked me if I had had any more medical testing. I told her that I hadn't. She replied, "You are saying that, based on your symptoms, you think it may be your thyroid."

"At this point, it might be my entire endocrine system that's not functioning properly," I answered.

"Well, your medical records say your thyroid is fine," she replied.

Hearing those repeated words set me off and caused me to have another episode of bursting in tears. Evidentially, the medical records were inconclusive. The weight of health professionals not listening to me and not giving legitimacy to my symptoms was aggressively breaking me down emotionally. The years of my health rapidly declining and no one investigating the root cause had left me bewildered and perplexed. I felt so alone and dejected. *How can I feel like something is physically wrong and no one else is picking this up?*

Despite how well the lab results said I was doing, my health continued to decline. Adamantly, I shared with the psychiatrist that returning to work would not be physically feasible for me. I advised her that if I did return it would be gravely detrimental to my health. I talked to her extensively about a medical leave of absence. I further explained that the lab tests did not show that a myriad of physical signs were alerting me that I was at a critical tipping point.

I had too many symptoms to deny the truth, regardless of the blood tests' results or the lack of a diagnosis. I wanted everyone to be on board with the seriousness of what I was sharing.

A few days later, I sat Lew down in the family room and said, "I have something important to tell you." From the look of fright on his face, he feared the worst. He knows all too well that I am a woman of few words. I don't waste my voice or my energy on frivolous speech. Therefore, when I said, "I have something to share with you," he leaned in to listen more closely to my every word.

"It's not that I do not want to return to work. I physically cannot. If I go back, it will not go well with me, and where will that leave you and Mikayla? I have to get the help I need."

"I understand," he said. "I have mixed emotions. I am happy that you decided to leave and pursue your health, but I'm afraid at the same time of where that will land us financially."

At that point, I didn't care about anything financial. When you come face to face with death, nothing other than life really matters.

Once I had a clear understanding with Lew, I contacted my doctor and the psychiatrist about my medical leave. In the mail, I received all the necessary paperwork for medical leave from Human Resources. I continued to work full time on improving my health while I sought out the root cause.

The Best News Ever

While on leave, I conducted a health experiment, and Lew joined me. We decided to eat raw fruits and vegetables for one month to see what kind of results we got. After thirty days, Lew lost fifteen pounds, but I lost no weight at all. This unscientific study further proved to me that my health was out of balance. We ate the same foods and got different results.

I remained on medical leave until the end of my contract year. When it was time to renew my contract, I declined. My symptoms were mounting, and I had no viable diagnosis. Therefore, it was in the best interest of my health to resign.

After my resignation, three years quickly passed, but I still did not have a diagnosis that matched my symptoms, although I continued to have blood work. Therefore, I called the doctor's office for an appointment for new lab work. Being home on medical leave for those three years gave me the much-needed rest my body and mind longed for. I was able to focus solely on my healing without the added responsibility of going to work every day. Finally, I was not as emotionally and physically exhausted as I had been while I was working.

Before I went to see the doctor, I researched ways to present my symptoms to the doctor so I could make the most of my appointment. I wanted to be sure that I followed a script he would understand so I could get my point across as accurately as I could without my emotions involved.

During the appointment, I pulled out my list of symptoms and spoke directly from it succinctly and matter-of-factly. He listened intently and called the nurse in to draw my blood. The next week, my lab results were in, and I was given an appointment to go over them. When I was in the examination room, the day felt like any other ordinary day. But by a long shot, it was not.

That day I was given the best news I had ever received. The moment I had longed for finally arrived. *Shabbat Shabbos* was on the horizon. Earlier in this chapter, I quoted from an online article: "A process must have an endpoint to give it meaning. If work never achieves a result, the work is foolish. ... So *Shabbos* teaches that all work must be directed to a goal."[20]

The doctor sat at his computer and read the entire contents of my lab report. Everything on the list he read out loud was very familiar to me, until he got to the point that showed I had elevated antibodies to my thyroid.

When he looked up at me to get my reaction, I had the biggest grin on my face. He continued, "You have Hashimoto Thyroiditis."

Every symptom I had been describing for years, starting with my irregular menstrual cycle from the age of thirteen up until that point became crystal clear as each symptom pointed directly to chronic thyroid disease. From the age of thirteen to age fifty-four, I had been begging health professionals to continue to probe to find the root cause of all the symptoms I had been experiencing.

This diagnosis opened the portal wide for me to begin my road to healing.

Normally I cry with each diagnosis, but this one was different. It was liberating because it defied medical gaslighting and the psychiatrist's report. Finally, I had a concrete reason for why my body was doing what it was doing—producing cysts, fainting, irregular periods, polycystic ovaries, anemia, headaches, fatty liver disease, low heart rate, high cholesterol, etc. In an instant, everything started to make sense to me.

What makes even more sense is that once I got my diagnosis, most everyone I have been in contact with that was diagnosed with Hashimoto Thyroiditis was also sent to see a psychiatrist. Although I should be dismayed by the length of time it took to get a real diagnosis and the toll that it took on my mental health trying to convince the medical establishment I was really sick, I look to my heavenly Father to avenge me.

Each medical hardship was strategically employed to be a companion to my weary soul and an ambassador of jubilation, all orchestrated under the tutelage of Christ to fix my eyes on him and his eternal plan versus the horrendous circumstances I had gone through. The lack of a proper diagnosis kept me running back to him for help, and he came through big time in his perfect timing. When God impressed upon my heart in prayer that he would give me *Shabbat Shabbos*, I believed him, and although I am weary from my searching, I still believe him now.

Chapter Seven

A Newfound Life Force

Let nothing which can be treated by diet be treated by other means.[21]

~ Maimonides

That wonderful and glorious day when I got the diagnosis of thyroid disease will forever be inscribed in my mind. Finally, all the health issues I had experienced for over four decades and purposefully tried to convey to the medical field started to make sense. My freedom came the week before Christmas 2015 … what a gift! Everything around our family was so festive and celebratory. This was the perfect time for a Christmas miracle.

Lew and I were invited to a party for food, fun, and fellowship, where our friends gathered for a pre-holiday celebration and gift exchange. Laughter and excitement filled the room where we all huddled. An unquestionably good time was had by all. After the presents were opened, everyone collected their personal belongings in preparation to go to their designated homes. Dinner with friends, more shopping, and waiting for out-of-town guests to arrive were some of the reasons the get-together had to be cut short.

Before the guests left, everyone clamored to get in their last-minute chatter, each out-talking the other. By flailing my hands in the air to get their attention, I caused everyone to stop what they were doing and look toward my direction. "Guys, before we go, I just want to quickly share that before coming here, I had a doctor's appointment, where I found out that I have an autoimmune disease called Hashimoto Thyroiditis."

At the sound of my words, impenetrable silence enveloped the room. The merriment turned to gloominess. Everyone stared at me. The news that I had been diagnosed with an unusual, unfamiliar-sounding disease during the most wonderful time of the year caused palpable, heartfelt sadness. I assured everyone that I was not the least disturbed by this new finding but, in fact, was overjoyed because I finally had a name for what I had been dealing with for so many years.

Once the veil of shock lifted, everyone fired questions at me. My goodness, their responses to me having an autoimmune disease were more overwhelming than the actual diagnosis. They wanted to know what my plans were for managing this disease. "Did the doctor put you on a diet restriction?" "Will you be taking medications to help with this?" "What does Hashimoto mean?"

The questions were unending, and the diagnosis was too new for me to give any concrete answers. I needed time to absorb and process this recent information. I could hardly wait to get home to research this disease and to investigate all that it entailed so I could discover which route was best for me. Until I received a diagnosis, I had not been equipped to answer any questions. Finally, when I was able to get a word in, I told everyone that I needed to research the disease before I could answer any more questions. Everyone agreed and said, "When you know, let us know."

Since the party ended at a reasonable hour, I had time to go home and search online databases and PubMed to find out what Hashimoto is and what would be my best approach to tackling it, in hopes of getting relief from my myriad of symptoms. My research, as I expected, yielded quite a bit of information and gave me a far greater understanding of my condition.

"Fight for Your Life!"

That Christmas, armed with the knowledge of Hashimoto's and the ramifications of a long delay in getting a diagnosis of this autoimmune disease, my family and I traveled to North Carolina for a reprieve and to spend the holidays with my cousins and their children. They have been up close and personal with me on this journey to wellness. They were always at the ready to see what they could do to help make life easier for me as I faced my giants. I could hardly wait to tell them that I finally got a long-awaited diagnosis. I could almost envision their responses and the look on their faces upon hearing this report.

During the five-hour car ride, a cloak of happiness enveloped me. There was a distinct awareness of newfound peace. Long-term sickness had shrouded my perspective for so long. Life always felt heavy and burdensome with no relief in sight. But during that holiday season, the weight of repeatedly rehearsing my symptoms to my medical team in an effort to find the root cause had been completely lifted off my shoulders. It had been a huge hardship to keep trying to explain something I was legitimately experiencing yet repeatedly being told that my labs didn't remotely match my explanation. It felt exhilarating to be free from that heavy responsibility. Doctors and patients are supposed to work in tandem. The burden of proof should not lie solely on patients to prove that they are really sick and need medical help.

While Lew drove us south, I sat back and observed passersby. Traveling on the interstate, I peered into random cars wondering if the people that I saw were also battling health challenges that they knew for certain existed but their validity was questioned by others. At rest stops, I wanted to talk to everyone I came in contact with. Something in me wanted to proclaim to everyone, "Fight for your life! Even when it takes a long time, maybe decades, do not give in to defeat. Be your own advocate. Don't let others silence you when you know in your heart what is true."

My audiences on the interstate and at the rest stops were just the beginning. Matter of fact, I wanted the entire world to know of my new findings and new freedom. I longed to share the importance of taking charge of your own health. "Never settle for anything less and do what's best for you" kept playing in my head on repeat. I couldn't bear to keep this news to myself.

Can you imagine carrying such a hefty load from age thirteen to age fifty-four, with increasing unsurmountable symptoms and no formal diagnosis that would validate what you continued to experience? In all those years, I could not even begin to imagine the damage done to my internal organs and tissues from the delay of not knowing specifically what to do. I'm so grateful that this prolonged disease did not cause my demise and that I am fully alive to share my story. As T. D. Jakes observed, "All of us have a story to tell. But not all of us survive to tell what happened and how we triumphed over the many tragedies that happened along the way."[22]

The lack of knowledge regarding the cause of my persistent symptoms resulted in the postponement of protocols and necessary treatment that could have alleviated my suffering. What a tremendous fight I had to endure for the sake of my health. But through divine grace, mercy, and strength, I was able to withstand the blows while I waited for further medical testing that unearthed this chronic, systemic disease along with the other four diseases discovered three months later. I've since learned, from several doctors, who themselves have been diagnosed with Autoimmune Thyroid Disease, that regular TSH thyroid blood tests can contradictorily show that the thyroid is normal. However, when experiencing multiple symptoms, a full thyroid panel consisting of Free T4, Free T3, Reverse T3, TSH, and thyroid antibodies must be ordered. The latter test probes much further than a TSH screening alone (Izabella Wentz PharmD, FASCP).[23]

All Hands on Deck

When we arrived at our destination in Charlotte, we jumped out of the car like two children and raced to ring the doorbell while Mikayla gathered her belongings from the back seat of the car. After quickly greeting everyone, we immediately unloaded our heavy suitcases out of the trunk of our vehicle and hoisted them onto the elevator to be transported to our upstairs bedroom. While the elevator rose to the second floor, Lew and I took the stairs. On the second floor, we waited for it to signal that we could safely open its doors. As soon as the light on the elevator button went off, we gathered our things and placed our belongings in our room. Without delay, we then hurried downstairs to tell everyone the great news.

Everyone organically gathered into the kitchen, where we all ended up standing around the periphery of the island. We formed a semicircle, far enough apart where each had their own personal space yet close enough to hear what everyone had to say.

Bursting with excitement, I blurted out, "It's been many years, but I fully know why I've felt unwell all these years."

Every eye was fastened on me, eagerly waiting for this great reveal.

"It's called Hashimoto. I have Hashimoto's," I said.

As I tried to explain the unfamiliar name, one cousin kept interrupting me. "Hashi who? Hashi who?" she repeated.

"It's a thyroid disease named after Dr. Hakaru Hashimoto, the Japanese doctor who discovered it," I answered.

The conversation continued as we reminisced about how many years it took to find out this important information and how my life had been spared in the interim. My family was so relieved to know that the report I had recently received did, in fact, closely resemble the symptoms I was having.

"You can't treat what you don't know," my cousin Dion added.

That evening, we stayed up past midnight talking and laughing about everything we could think of. I could hardly sleep because I was bursting with joy and excitement. Throughout the night, I continued to check the clock to be sure that the time was moving toward morning so I could share more of what I had learned.

The next morning, I told my family that the biggest discovery I had made so far through my research was the effect that gluten has on the body in general and the thyroid in particular. In the docuseries called "Betrayal: The Autoimmune Disease Solution They're Not Telling You," Dr. Tom O'Bryan, the world's leading gluten expert, specifically talks about how gluten has a direct link to autoimmune disease. He makes it very clear that gluten must be eliminated from the body immediately.[24]

We spent a considerable amount of time that morning trying to figure out which foods would be best for me to eat in order to alleviate my current symptoms and avoid new ones. It was so refreshing and fun to see all hands on deck to ensure that nothing bad from that moment forward could touch me. Everyone was so protective and caring. Each item of food was held up, followed by a firing of questions: "Dawn, can you eat this?" and "Can you eat this?" and "How about this?" For the remainder of our time there,

I ate everything I wanted, but I strictly abstained from foods I thought could cause possible inflammation.

From the onset of my diagnosis, I stopped eating gluten, eggs, dairy, and processed sugar. Despite my self-imposed food restrictions, Christmas 2015 was the best holiday for me in a very long time because having a diagnosis stimulated hope. In my mind's eye, I was already imagining what future holidays would look like for me.

Time passed quickly. In the blink of an eye, our vacation was over. The planned activities, such as going to the movies and playing archery, made the family fun times go even faster. The day we were to leave to go back home, the family gathered once again in the kitchen, where I shared with them that the food choices I had made over the weekend felt pretty good. Leaving out the inflammatory foods proved to be quite beneficial. Straying from what I normally ate and tweaking my food preferences did not feel burdensome at all. Quite frankly, I did not miss the foods I averted.

A New Dietary Regimen

While we were on the subject of food, I further announced that I wanted to continue what I had done in that short time frame and make this way of eating a total lifestyle change to further test its impact on my health. This was quite exciting for me. I had never done anything like this before. The variety of my food or the lack thereof has always been routine. I ate the same things repeatedly. Making this type of change further solidified that it's my body and I need to experiment to see what works best for me.

I was armed with newfound strength to explore the possibilities of bringing my body back to health. In light of this, I disclosed that I was contemplating a water fast when I returned home. My main objective for fasting was to make every effort to clear out the old, harmful foods, to give my body a rest from digestion, and to allow it time to clean out my tissues and cells from the foods I had eaten that did not agree with my system. According to Philippus Paracelsus, "Fasting is the greatest remedy. The physician within."[25] The excitement of fasting ran through my mind during my entire stay. I was constantly thinking about it. I was so eager to get on with restoring my health that it raised in me a level of excitement I had never experienced.

Many people are not aware of the power of hope. In one diagnosis, I went from impossible to possible, from despair to hope, from "you will always be sick" to "you can heal," from "no one is hearing me" to "everyone is hearing me."

The urge to fast was quite strong, sometimes overwhelming. While Lew slept, I lay in bed and played out scenarios in my head of what fasting would be like. *What could I expect? Will I get weaker? Will I be hungry? How many days can I fast?* While these questions bombarded my mind, my heart raced with adventure because I knew that great things were happening and that I was in full charge.

After a night of contemplation, I outlined to my family the next morning how I wanted to start and end my fast. My goal was to try this fast for seven days, but with the stipulation and promise that the moment I felt any discomfort I would stop the water fast— even if that meant ending my fast after only one day of being on it.

It was important to me that everyone present was privy to my plans because they were always there for me throughout this entire journey. I was not about to leave them out. They had heard the bad news for so many years; now it was time for them to hear the good news of a plan well thought out regarding my new and improved health goals. I welcomed their feedback because I wanted to be certain that my elation for desperately wanting to heal did not cloud my sensible judgment in any way. Everyone seemed to be in agreement with my intentions, and they know me well enough to know that I exercise common sense. Unanimously they said, "Take it one day at a time."

Excitement Beyond Belief

When we arrived back home, the holiday season was coming to a close. More than two weeks had passed since I had changed my eating habits, and I felt better than I had ever felt. A new year was beginning, a time when most of the world makes new resolutions. My diagnosis could not have come at a better time. I perspicaciously knew the diagnosis was not the final answer. I felt that there was much more I had to learn about Hashimoto's and its effects on the body: What triggers it? What is the root cause? What foods should I eat? What foods should I avoid? None of that knowledge was evident or in plain sight. As if searching for hidden treasure, I had to actively participate in diligently seeking it out. January was the perfect month for me to take on a new challenge toward healing and wholeness.

The concept of fasting was not new to me. My mom had fasted upwards of forty days at a time for spiritual reasons. However, prior to my fast, I had never heard of anyone fasting for one's health. Fortunately, I discovered tons of books and resources available to help anyone who wants to integrate fasting into their healing regiment. Since I've become aware of fasting as a means to accelerate my healing, I am now cognizant of many others who incorporate fasting for health reasons. Now that I've tried it, it seems that the idea of fasting as a means of promoting health is found everywhere, even on all social media platforms. More people than I ever expected are fasting their way to health.

Fasting is not just for humans; animals fast instinctively. One day, I observed that my dog, a bichon frise, had stopped eating because he did not feel well. I'm told that observing what goes on in nature is the best way to know what we humans should also be doing. I've watched my dog Spark, without any physical manifestation that he was sick, avoid food for days. I became conscious of what he was doing once I started fasting. He would not even go near his food bowl until he felt better. Wow! That was an eye-opener for me.

As I was fasting, I wanted to learn everything I could to keep me focused and motivated, especially since everyone else in my household was eating. I devoured the book *The Miracle of Fasting: Proven Throughout History for Physical, Mental, & Spiritual Rejuvenation* by Paul C. and Patricia Bragg. It states that "the miracle of fasting aids in flushing deadly poisons from the body. When we fast (stop eating) all the Vital Force that has been used to convert food into energy and body tissue is now being used to flush poisons from the body!"[26] In a nutshell, this was the whole motivation of my fast. I wanted to flush out anything in my body that was causing disease. Reading that book highly inspired me to continue.

Fasting was much more beneficial than I anticipated. After seven full days of water only, I completed my fast. The results were far beyond anything I could have imagined. Like a person who is madly in love, I recall feelings of butterflies fluttering in my stomach and excitement beyond belief. This new relationship with fasting was the beginning of our long journey together. Each day, I basked in the notion that I was evicting poisons and allowing my body time and space to replace old cells with new ones. Wanting to experience that euphoria again and again, I could hardly wait for the next day. For me, there was no hunger at all during my fast. Excitement was my predominant feeling, sending waves of endorphins throughout my body. I felt energized, cleansed, happy, and expectant. These emotions had been nonexistent for most of my life; they had been buried deep in the crevices of sickness and despair. Fasting allowed them to rise to the surface and break forth like budding flowers facing the sun, leaving in their emergence a greater tenacity for more.

In view of this, I wanted to hold tightly to the ecstasy that I partook of during my fast. I refused to let this newfound exhilaration wane. I enjoy food. It gives me great comfort and delight in addition to nourishing my body. However, once I also experienced the bliss of fasting, I wanted it to be an integral part of me. Just like I ate regularly, I also wanted to fast regularly to maintain those newly found feelings with the possibility of permanently increasing them.

Return to Mother Nature

As my fast came to an end, I knew that I would have to slowly reintroduce food into my body to feed and nourish my cells. Any type of fasting must be done wisely and sensibly. At the end of my fast, I decided that I wanted to figure out ways to sustain this ecstatic feeling. I felt revived, clean, and happy. What could I do to sustain this newfound life force? I pondered that question repeatedly.

I decided to try eating just raw foods. No cooking, no sugar, no salt, and no oils—just raw food as found in Mother Nature. To me, this was the next best thing for me after fasting. I wanted to supply my body with all the life force nature offered without being hungry or counting calories.

Like with fasting, I did not put a time limit on eating this way. I left it up to my body to tell me when to stop and start. I took it one day at a time. Each day indescribable things began to happen in my body. In addition to inwardly feeling the best I had ever felt, within months, what was happening internally began to manifest outwardly. For instance, rashes I had on my armpits began to disappear, the skin on my face became clearer with less acne, and small skin tags on my neck dropped off unexpectedly.

From witnessing all these wonderful healings happening spontaneously, I probed further to see if any changes occurred in other areas where I have always longed to be different. Sure enough, I saw other changes taking place. For instance, my middle finger used to be bent in a forty-five-degree angle due to rheumatoid arthritis. My holistic doctor had been so afraid it would remain that way permanently and eventually the other fingers would follow suit. That finger is now flattened and straight.

With these kinds of results, sliding into a raw diet was not difficult at all. Matter of fact, I wanted to continue because I wanted to see more results like these. There was so much raw food for me to choose from. Not once did I focus on what I was missing out on. My eyes were fixed on all the good I was gaining. I had a lot of work to do in my body, and the method I had chosen was agreeable. I didn't know how long all these changes would be in effect, but I wanted to go as long as I could to see what would happen next.

When I started to see the changes, I began to place checkmarks near the list of healings I was believing for and working toward. Sickness had permeated me for a very long time, leaving me tired and depleted. I had to allow my physical being time and space to go to work and do its repair. "When you eat foods picked fresh from nature, and eat them without cooking or processing them, the high electromagnetic energy of that food is transferred to your body and its cells."[27] I knew I needed lots of energy because for years I had lacked energy. Raw food was my best choice for obtaining energy, which would allow my body room to heal. "As homo sapiens, we need at least 6000 to 7000 angstroms of systemic energy at all times to even begin to smile, no less to be happy and healthy."[28] I ate foods reminiscent of those in the biblical garden of Eden, where my ancestors were created to eat, live, and work. I made sure each day I had a bounty of food. I ate plenty. My food choices consisted of fruits, vegetables, nuts, and seeds. I ate whatever I wanted and whenever I desired. No rules, no restrictions. Just freedom. No counting calories or looking at the clock to dictate when to eat. I ate intuitively when I was hungry.

Concierge Doctors

After my weeklong fast followed by eating raw energetic food, I was motivated to venture into something new. Within three months of my Hashimoto Thyroiditis diagnosis, I added concierge doctors to my team. I've learned from having extensive blood work that it takes approximately three months to see notable changes in my chemistry. I chose a concierge doctor because I wanted to be in a practice where I could get the best care possible. I wanted a doctor who was not limited by time but would be willing to take as much time as needed to access my health and make recommendations. Since I was making new and drastic changes, I wanted new doctors. Concierge doctors offer premium services to their patients. With this type of medical service, I was given 24/7 access, which included having my doctors' cell phone numbers, same day appointments if I needed them, and doctor visits that lasted as long as necessary.

Eating raw food and fasting allowed me to see notable changes inwardly and outwardly. Therefore, I wanted a full and extensive lab work-up along with specialized follow-up to delve into the changes occurring internally. I needed a physician who would listen to my health needs and not dismiss any of my symptoms nor be constrained to order only tests the insurance companies allowed. I wanted to be treated as a whole person, not the sum of my parts. I wanted a physician who understood autoimmune disease and its effects on the body as a whole, not just the place where it was found. For example, I was diagnosed with Hashimoto Thyroiditis, which is primarily thyroid disease. Yet the small, butterfly-shaped thyroid located in the front of my neck produces hormones that are responsible for my body's metabolic rate, heart, digestion, muscles, brain, mood, bones, and many other areas I'm not aware of. With all that I had gone through, I needed tender loving care (TLC). Even though Hashimoto Thyroiditis affects the thyroid directly, its effects are felt systemically throughout the body.

During my first visit at the concierge doctor's office, I took note that the atmosphere was warm and welcoming. The doctors and staff seemed more like friends than a medical team. Their genuine care for their patients was evident, and I experienced that genuine care firsthand. Before my visit, I filled out all my medical history online, paving the way for my new doctor and me to talk face-to-face about my health goals and aspirations. I was in awe of the amount of time they had taken to get to know me and my family personally. My concierge doctors did not sit in a big chair across from me like other doctors had. Instead, they sat on the sofa with me as if we were in their family room having a visit.

The office was airy with well-appointed furniture and medical accoutrements. Before my conversation with the doctor, I was taken to a room in the back where the phlebotomist was given a detailed sheet indicating which labs were to be ordered. This was the most extensive lab work I had ever had. I had been accustomed to getting general lab work such as my cholesterol levels, basic thyroid, kidney function, etc. However, this fasting blood test consisted of a whole lot more. Although I came to these doctors with my previous labs, which showed that I had Hashimoto's, they wanted to retest me anyway.

I'm glad they did because the previous tests were three months old. I could hardly wait to see what effects my new lifestyle changes were producing in my blood. My doctors ordered labs for a blood count test which detects anemia, infections, and leukemia along with a full panel thyroid test that includes TSH, Free T4, Free T3, Reverse T3, TPO Antibodies and TG Antibodies, extensive autoimmune testing, a cholesterol test with particle count, and a blood test for liver, kidney, and cancer. In addition, I was given a food allergy test and a stool test to detect parasites and bacterial overgrowth.

How Do I Conquer All of This?

To see my lab results, I was given the website login and username to access their in-house patient portal where my lab results and the doctors' comments would be stored. Through this portal, I am able to set up subsequent appointments. A week later, I received an automatic email stating that my lab work was in and I should book my next appointment through the portal. I logged into the portal for a quick peek at my results, but the report was so detailed, I definitely needed a linguist to help me to decipher its meaning.

I was able to secure an appointment the next day. At this visit, the doctor and I sat at a small table with two folders placed in front of each chair. One folder was for my records, and one was for my doctor. The doctor went over the full report with a fine-tooth comb and explained every minute detail to me. While following along, I listened as my doctor read aloud the other autoimmune diseases that had been picked up in my recent lab work.

When I heard the words Hashimoto Thyroiditis, I said to myself, "Okay, I know what that is. But wait!" She kept reading off the list: rheumatoid arthritis ... lupus ... Raynaud's disease ..."

I gasped. What? Wait a minute. Are you saying I have all of these? Did these really show up in my blood work?

I sat there with my hand over my mouth. Years of my broken life flooded before me. Tears streamed down my face. I began to wish that my mother was still alive because I needed so desperately to let her know that I had found the reason for all my physical pain and suffering. I felt the weight of how wrongly I had been treated. I was prepared to tackle Hashimoto's, but I did not feel equipped to handle all the other diseases, too, especially knowing that each autoimmune disease affects different parts of the body and does different types of cellular and tissue damage.

My world began to spin. How do I conquer all of this? Where do I start? How many specialists will I have to see? There are five autoimmune diseases, so I will need at least five different doctors.

As the tears flowed down my cheeks, my doctor reached over and held my hand while she displayed a reassuring smile. She said, "We are going to take good care of you."

As we continued to talk, she said, "Whenever someone is diagnosed with Hashimoto's and has had it for quite some time without being treated, you can expect there to be more autoimmune to follow." That's why she had run such extensive blood work. She went on to say, "Every autoimmune has a trigger. Has anything happened to you recently that caused you to feel worse than ever?"

"Yes," I said, hot tears streaming down my face. "My mother died."

The doctor got up from her chair, hugged me, and said, "We are going to get to the bottom of this. You have a solid team now."

Although I cried my eyeballs out, I left the doctors' office with a greater determination to fight for my life. I was grateful for the support and help I was receiving, but I knew that due to the extent of damage these autoimmune diseases had wreaked on my health, I needed to take the helm and be at the forefront of my healing.

Yes, I have a strong team, but I must be the general manager. No one knows me like I do. I had to take back my power that had been involuntarily relinquished to doctors over the years. I'm in charge of the state of affairs regarding my health. No one is responsible for my health except me.

Two Prophetic Dreams

In the days that followed, I continued to pray for answers to overcome all these diseases. I steadfastly evoked the help from the One who created me. A couple of years before any of these diagnoses, I had two very poignant dreams. I rarely remember my dreams. Therefore, the ones I do remember stay indelibly printed on my heart and mind. When a dream leaves that kind of lasting impression upon me, I innately know that it has a greater meaning for a later date or time. Therefore, upon awakening from any remembered dream, I usually type it in my notes on my iPad along with a description and the date so it's easily accessible when I need to refer to it.

These dreams were very telling. Matter of fact, looking back, they were prophetic in nature, pointing to exactly what lies ahead for me. At the time of my dreams, the meaning was hidden from me. However, in light of my experiences, it has been revealed that these dreams were a significant and pertinent part of my journey, indicating what I'll need to do to eradicate disease in my body.

The first recurring dream takes place in a very large school building that stretches the span of ten city blocks. It has an east wing and a west wing with several floors. In the dream, I am sitting at a student's desk, taking copious notes and highly engaged in learning, but no teacher stands in front of me. I sit there for the duration of the school day, never taking lunch or any other breaks in between. I have no need for food at that time. All I want to do is sit there and learn. When classes end and it is time for me to go home, I have difficulty finding my way out of the building. Therefore, I go from classroom to classroom in this massive building looking for someone to give me directions on how to get out of the building. Only one other person is in the building. Finally, I locate that person and ask, "Where is the exit?" After receiving detailed directions, I still cannot find the exit. I am left wandering the entire building looking for a way out. That's how the dream always ends.

Upon awakening, I pondered the dream's meaning. Unlike Joseph, the son of Jacob in the Bible, I haven't been given the gift of interpreting dreams. However, looking back on what I've gone through and where it has brought me today, I've concluded that this recurring dream meant I was going to be faced with decisions that would require an extensive amount of learning, hence the large school building. And I also surmise that the reason I could not find the exit was because I was not able to leave the school because I had more learning to acquire. Although the school day ended in my dream, that didn't mean my learning had ended. Once I gain the knowledge I need, then I will be able to find my way to the exit of the school building.

The second recurring dream I have is similar in nature yet different. In this dream, I am traveling alone on what appears to be the West Coast. I have no cell phone or purse with me. My feet are the only mode of transportation available. In my quest to get home, I start on my journey and soon arrive at a beautiful, picturesque neighborhood lined with majestic, tall trees. I watch a breathtaking sunset as I walk. It is almost dusk, and I am eager to find my way back home before the day fades into darkness. As I walk past one of the houses, I see a Caucasian man tending to his flowers and shrubbery on the side of his yard facing the street. Since I am traveling alone, seeing someone in the neighborhood brings me comfort. I am not alone. When I come into his peripheral view, he glances at me, yet quickly returns his attention to what he is doing. As I continue, I reach the end of his street. In front of me is a vast body of water, which appears to be an ocean.

With no way to cross the water, I turn around to go back the way I came, hoping to find another route home. As I walk up the hill past the side of the house where the man is tending to his yard, he looks up and begins to run his hand down the side of his house, telling me how the salt water from the ocean is corroding the side of his house. I long to engage in conversation because I am by myself, but my main objective is to find my way home before dark. Therefore, I am polite yet dismissive. I wave at him to acknowledge his comment, and I keep walking. When I have walked a few feet away, I hear a well-defined noise, which causes me to turn around to see what is going on. The man is waving his arms, as if he is shooing something from his yard. He repeatedly says, "Go," as he continues to wave. Finally, I see an exceptionally large owl perched on one of the tree branches in the man's yard. The owl's colors are noticeably vibrant and distinct, but his markings camouflage him because they match his environment.

Each time I awoke from this dream, the tremendous size of the owl replayed constantly in my mind. I shared the dream with Lew and told him that I believed the dream meant something is getting ready to occur in my life that is going to require great wisdom and insight.

My mom's favorite admonition was "Be wise as an owl." Both recurring dreams happened long before I was ever diagnosed. One dream deals with learning; the other dream deals with wisdom. They make much more sense to me today than they did when I dreamt them. I strongly believe these dreams are a part of the hidden messages needed for my healing journey. Even today, their meaning has not yet been totally revealed; their significance is still unfolding.

Chapter Eight

Metamorphosis

The pain of recovery is often greater than the pain of injury, but healing is worth it.[29]

~ Christine Caine

In the following years, those recurring dreams proved invaluable. Their meaning came into fuller fruition, not when I was first diagnosed but rather when I searched for unconventional ways to restore my body to its original design. I longed for education and wisdom—no small feat.

The beginning days of healing were my honeymoon phase. Everything seemed so new and fresh. As I ate raw food exclusively during the first full year after the diagnoses, my body aggressively began to slough off things I never even imagined could dwell inside a viable human being. I became aware of this type of deep penetrating cleansing during the first three months of eating raw. For example, one day after I finished my lunch, I felt an urge to go to the bathroom and, with no effort at all, out popped this weird looking specimen that resembled a fish with one eye. I had just signed on with concierge doctors, and since I have 24/7 access to them, I took a picture of the specimen, then called them right away to schedule an appointment so I could show them what my body had expelled. This was perfect timing because they had recently run tons of labs on me, and I wanted to see how the specimen fit in with the lab results.

Throughout my life, I have had a sensitive stomach. The least little thing I see or smell can make me nauseous days on end. Surprisingly, during my healing journey, I've been given a special gift of grace to not be squeamish or fearful about what I've seen coming out of me. The years behind me have proven that I have toughened up. Let's be clear, though. This toughness is for me only. I can't bear to look at the excrement of others. When I went to the bathroom, the unusual swish sound attracted my attention and made me inquisitive. This thing came out so fast, I didn't feel anything abnormal. When I looked in the toilet, the water was clear—perfect for taking a picture to show my doctors.

Nothing else came out with the odd specimen. It swam alone in the toilet bowl's clear water. I could hardly wait to see what my concierge doctor would say it was. When I got to her office, she was standing at the front desk waiting for me. The first thing I asked was, "Do you have a weak stomach? Because I need to show you what came out of me."

When I pulled up my photos, she took one look and said, "I've never seen anything like that in my life." Her answer was honest but disappointing. I wanted to know the name of what was being expelled from my body.

In the following days, similar occurrences happened daily. I did not have a name for these specimens either, so every time something odd came out, I said to Lew, "Guess what? Sickness and disease came out of me again today."

Lew usually responded, "Oh, one of those creature-looking things came out again?"

Expelling Biofilm

It took months of researching and connecting with people on social media who were on a similar healing journey before I learned the actual name of what I was expelling out of me—biofilm. "Microbial biofilms can colonize on medical devices and human tissues, and their role in microbial pathogenesis is now well established. ... This multicellular aggregated form of microbial growth confers a remarkable resistance to killing by antimicrobials and host defenses, leading biofilms to cause a wide range of subacute or chronic infections that are difficult to eradicate."[30]

I also started visiting a new primary care physician (PCP) who believed in employing both a conventional and holistic approach to her patients. I wanted answers to what was coming out of my system. I took that same picture to her and asked the same question. "Do you have a weak stomach?"

After viewing my pictures, she was silent. She left me in the examining room, and later came back with a printed computer paper. On it was the name of a supplement she wanted me to take right away. She immediately prescribed that I go to my local health food store and purchase Serrapeptase, a proteolytic enzyme that would break down the matrix of the biofilm without causing any harm to its host—my body.

I couldn't believe I was the host of biofilm. When the doctor told me, I felt disgusted and violated that some creature had invaded and permeated my body unbeknownst to me. The high astringent food and clean diet were driving out the biofilm.

This new doctor didn't let on that she knew what the specimen was, but thankfully, she knew what to do. I'm not certain which organs housed this biofilm, but I do know that for one year straight, it was ejected daily from my body. I kept a flashlight in my bathroom so I could clearly see the abnormalities leaving my temple.

Witnessing my body expel foreign matter marked the beginning of many physical signs that confirmed for me how sick I was. Many people may dispute that these things can exist in a human. However, I will never be held hostage by someone's opinion when I have an experience—not one that I welcomed but an experience nonetheless.

As this biofilm was leaving my body, some specimens seemed too large to pass, which sometimes caused excruciating pain. The first one came out so easily I thought expulsions would always be that way, but the subsequent ones were quite difficult. The worst part was when one got stuck in my colon and caused considerable discomfort. I had to walk around with it in me until it was ready to come out on its own. Over time I tried to force it out, but that was too painful. For hours, I lay on my bathroom floor, praying and crying and asking God to alleviate the pain and help this thing to pass safely.

"I Just Want to Be Free!"

Thankfully, one of my cousins introduced me to enemas. She specifically said that when someone makes a drastic diet change like I did, that old mess has to come out. So, she walked me through the steps of how to perform an enema.

With my new dietary changes and lifestyle, I became unusually aware of my body and its functions. Just like before the diagnoses, I knew something was wrong with me when others chose not to believe me. I now operate in a higher level of awareness. But this time, I'm not looking for anyone to validate my experiences. On my raw food diet, I started doing enemas once a week to ensure that all the old matter was thoroughly expelled.

The amount that came out was beyond belief. It was shocking even to me. I kept asking, "Where is my small frame housing all of this stuff?" Every day even more wanted to come out. I stayed tied to a bathroom. Leaving my house was nearly impossible. Things were coming out of my system so fast that I couldn't keep up. *Did I go too fast in detoxing? Should I have only fasted a few days and not engaged in a weeklong fast? Should I stop eating raw and incorporate some cooked food to slow this process?* These questions swarmed in my mind.

Some days I felt like the biofilm was lodged in my colon and not even an enema could remove it. That's when I became frightened, thinking that if the enema didn't help to remove it, then I had no other recourse to get the mass out. On many days, I felt as if the biofilm was going to be permanently lodged in my colon. I began to have panic attacks. One enema on any given day led to another, then another.

"I just want to be free," I screamed.

Having foreign matter stuck in my colon and being acutely aware of it made me very afraid. This was cause for great concern. I cried out in fear and terror. Imagine a mass protruding from your rectum that is causing great distress, yet you cannot pass it. It won't go back up, and it won't come out. What a bad predicament I found myself in!

As my body continued its internal cleansing, the effects of removing matter that had been embedded in my body for years began to take an emotional toll on me. This was not a one-time occurrence. This happened every day for years. The panic attacks became more frequent. With no relief in sight, my emotions became too fragile to handle the onslaught of embedded debris that was being stirred up daily in my bloodstream and in my body. "Endotoxin, if not eliminated daily from your colon through Gentle Daily Cleansing, can and will be absorbed into the bloodstream causing inflammation to the weakest parts of the body or throughout the whole body."[31]

Panic Attacks

The anxiety attacks were fierce, and they always presented themselves without warning. I tried to calm myself from the onslaught of these attacks through prayer, meditation, infrared sauna sessions, reading the Scriptures, and taking daily walks. Using one of my relaxing techniques, I decided to give myself an in-home pampering session one day. I took out my foot bath and poured one cup of Epsom salts in it, along with a few drops of lavender for fragrance and a calming effect. I added warm water from my teakettle. For ambience, I played some spa music through the television in my family room, which is adjacent to my kitchen. I sat at my kitchen table where everything I needed was on hand. Nearby was my soft foot towel, my iPad, and my cordless phone. I placed my feet in the warm bath, folded my hands behind my head, and gently leaned my head back to peer through the skylight to soak in the beauty of the tall trees gently swaying in the sunny blue sky.

Approximately ten minutes into my foot soak and meditation, my skylight disappeared, and the twenty-foot ceilings closed in on me. I started hyperventilating and having extreme heart palpitations. My tan-colored walls became gray. Everything seemed to be swirling in black and white. Minutes passed and I did not know where I was. My surroundings no longer looked familiar. I tried to center my emotions by breathing in through my nose and out through my mouth but to no avail. Each breath seemed as if it would be my last.

Instinctively, I knew I needed to call for help. *If someone doesn't get here quickly, I won't make it. My breathing is getting more sporadic.* I prayed, "Lord, help me. I'm scared. I don't want to die. I want to live."

I quickly removed my feet from the foot bath because having them there made me feel even more confined. Remembering the phone was on the table, I picked it up to call Lew for help, but I could not recall his number. At that moment, I interpreted forgetting his number as a sign that he was gone and I was in the world all alone. A feeling of hopelessness overcame me. *The walls are now closing in. I feel trapped!*

I needed to run out of my house to be where the atmosphere was more open, but I realized I was wearing only a T-shirt and my underwear. With water dripping from my feet, I ran with purpose and determination to my freezer, opened up the ice maker, and grabbed handfuls of ice to shove down my shirt and underwear in an effort to shock myself out of the awful panic attack.

By the time I managed to place several handfuls of ice cubes down my clothes, Lew entered the kitchen from the garage door and found me sobbing hysterically over the kitchen sink with my clothes soaking wet from the ice cubes melting on my shivering body.

I will never forget the look of horror on his face. He had barely closed the kitchen door when he ran to me and held me tightly while he called on our Lord and Savior. I heard him sternly say, "Lord please deliver my wife." He stayed with me until the panic attack subsided and did not return to work until he knew for certain that I was okay. The scene that he walked into left him feeling powerless.

"Your Brain Is Firing Too Much"

Those severe, unwelcomed panic attacks continued for two years, preventing me from going in tight spaces, riding rides at amusement parks, getting into small cars, and being in crowds. The type of fear I felt that day was the kind my ancestors experienced during a fight-or-flight response when they had to run to safety from a saber-toothed tiger chasing after them.

Lew surmised that these attacks were brought on because my body was going through a healing crisis coupled with my subconscious and conscious desperation to be made whole. He gave me a great strategy to diffuse the attacks before they started.

He said, "Whenever you remotely begin to feel overwhelmed, get up and walk away from the situation—whether it's internal or external."

Weeks later, I found another doctor to add to my team. I wanted to talk to as many medical professionals as I could to let them know that we have to take autoimmune very seriously. These are chronic diseases that have systemic effects throughout the body. When I spoke to him for an hour over the phone, I wanted it to be clear that, at this point, I was only interested in seeing doctors who either have Hashimoto's or who have extensive training in this chronic disease. He went to great lengths to assure me that he had special training in Hashimoto's.

I've learned that all chronic diseases are multifactorial, which means nothing happens in isolation. My other autoimmune diseases were prevalent, and I wanted to be cured from them all, but when talking to health practitioners, I mainly emphasized help for Hashimoto's because unlike the other autoimmune diseases, my Hashimoto's had advanced to stage five by the time I was diagnosed. "Stage one is genetic predisposition, Stage two is Immune Cell Infiltration of the Thyroid Gland, Stage three is Subclinical Hypothyroidism, Stage four is Overt Hypothyroidism, Stage five is progression to other Autoimmune Disorders."[32] Knowing that the misdiagnosis caused me to advance to stage five, I wanted immediate help to lessen the damage and stop further progression as quickly as possible.

The day of my appointment I was given extensive testing that I had not been given before. After completing the tests, the doctor told me, "Your brain is firing too much, which caused the anxiety attacks and the heart palpitations, which is a direct symptom of Hashimoto's." My entire body was in turmoil on the inside, although I looked calm on the outside. He also stated that "your left hemisphere is not responding well to the diagnostic testing I am administering." Therefore, he took an x-ray of my head and neck to rule out any hidden problems.

Fear had me up all night praying that nothing was found on the x-ray, especially since years prior I had had the incident at work where my blood platelets seemed to be sticking together, which caused a popping sound in my head. I was relieved when the test found nothing unusual in my head and neck.

Eager to get information on how to handle the masses of foreign matter coming out of me, I divulged to him that I was on a raw diet, which was causing my body to cleanse at a fast pace releasing biofilm, cholesterol stones, gallstones, and lots of fat. Like the other doctors, he had not heard of anyone expelling biofilms. I had to continue to stay focused and determined to try whatever I could to give my body what it needed to continue its cleansing work. The hardened crusted matter that my body was releasing was a clear sign that it too wanted to be free from the things I had ingested that did not add value to my health.

Helpful Summits on Health

I do not know how this happens, but when you search diligently for knowledge, I believe that no matter how long it takes, it will come to you. Mine took over three decades, but thankfully, it came. One day, in my inbox was an email inviting me to sign up for an online Women's Wellness Summit. I was intrigued by the title. I signed up and attended this seven-day summit via my computer in the comfort of my home.

This summit was a gift from God. The panel of experts spoke about health-related issues I had never been exposed to. Each woman shared individual stories of how, with the right care, her body was able to heal and return to homeostasis. That was the best news I had ever heard. This summit brought hope beyond measure. Three months later, I received another email inviting me to attend a Healing Hashimoto's Summit. These summits were so timely, and I wondered why I had not heard about them through any of my doctors or my research.

Later I learned that my name was starting to get circulated among medical doctors who left their conventional practices to start holistic practices because they wanted to get away from the demands of the insurance companies and they wanted the liberty to really take time to help and care for their patients. All these invitations came at the time I needed them most. I knew this was divine destiny. Everything was being aligned for me to have a sure footing in taking on the massive task of restoring my health.

At the Hashimoto's Summit I first heard the words, "You can heal." Those three words changed the trajectory of my life. I was given supernatural divine wisdom to navigate this bumpy, winding road to complete wholeness. When I decided to embark on the journey of regenerating my body, little did I know about the pain and suffering I would have to endure to move my body from a chronic acidosis state to a regenerative state. Each layer of disease that was removed brought its own set of challenges. It seemed that as I took one step forward, I was pushed three steps backward. *What is this? I thought healing was going to be easy. I thought suffering was behind me.*

I was blindsided. This path to healing is not for the faint of heart. It takes tenacity and persistence to heal at the cellular level. It requires lots of praying, biohacking, experimenting, sleepless nights, and fortitude to stick with the plan until you get the results you always wanted. I had to do what I had never done before to get the results I had never had.

Although I had the names of my illnesses, I didn't know the extent of my illness until I saw what was coming out of me. Expelling foreign matter painted the whole picture for me. It revealed stories untold. My body was a wasteland of sorts. It had degenerated to a place of internal hardness. There was no flow. It was filled with stones, cysts, scar tissue, mucus, and parasites. No nutrients were able to come in, and no toxins were going out.

With the onslaught of my body getting into balance and releasing years of toxic sludge, I was drained and depleted. Many days, I did not think I could physically or mentally go on. Although healing was taking place, my body was also taking a beating, which in turn affected my mental health. During the intense hardship of going through the healing process, my body had become a metaphorical battlefield, and my sanity was its casualty. My emotional equilibrium was off kilter due to the intense struggle to heal. I was going through a physical metamorphosis, and my mind and my soul needed to be strong enough to endure the vast changes.

My greatest downfall was my expectation of what healing looked like. Healing is not linear. It's up and down, zigzag, circular, peaks and valleys. Healing is messy. I had to be broken down to be rebuilt so I could be stronger for my next level. I had to excavate and unearth the real me who was buried under the weight of systemic acidosis called sickness and disease.

Living in the Spirit Realm

When my body hurts every day, it automatically keeps me connected to my sensory/soulish realm. I work hard to elevate my spirit because living in the spirit realm is where I want to be. It's the essence of who I really am. That part of me is what I want to grow and mature. It's in that space I can live like I was designed and created to be.

I've always been passionate about helping people to be confident that God has a unique plan for them. While my tests and trials grew, I held on tightly, albeit with bloody hands and white knuckles, to my confidence that God has a plan for me. That truth was trying to slip from my grasp. The hardest moments were when I felt like I didn't know what else to do to move forward. Sometimes God strategically led me for quite a while, and then he got quiet. I felt lost. Yes, lost is a real daunting place. The scariest part for me was the amount of time I was allowed to remain lost and how I was able to physically feel every emotion associated with being lost and the deep longing and intense desire to be found. I needed constant divine intervention.

Nothing in life prepared me for the hardest moments. The trauma of unending sickness left me with a lot of questions. I questioned my salvation, my sanity, my purpose, and my position. I don't understand how I survived it all. I was emotionally unprepared for the onslaught of what was being released from my body. I was already fragile due to the fact that I had been sick all my life.

I entered into detoxification on the heels of yet another unfavorable doctor's report. Hashimoto's was enough to handle, and then all these other autoimmune diseases came aboard. I was still reeling from that news when I decided to clean up my diet and fast. The raw astringent foods began to work and loosen the hardened matter that had taken up residence in me. So, when my body began to shake loose the hardened debris, my emotions ran wild. This went on for years. Detoxification at this magnitude causes unforeseen emotions. No wonder health healers sternly express that when you go to this level, it is imperative that you work with those who are trained to walk you through what Saint John of the Cross called the "dark night of the soul."[33]

A Great Dumping

Emotions emerged that I didn't know I had. The ones that surfaced were sadness, fear, dread, anxiousness, timidity, and uncertainty. Surprisingly, I also experienced what it was like for my body to detox the few pharmaceuticals I had taken in my younger years. With each bite of healthy life-giving food, every cell began to be transformed. I call it "a great dumping." Once I removed the foods that didn't agree with my body's chemistry, my body went "for broke" and waged an all-out war to rid itself of anything that didn't serve it.

I can't explain this in any scientific terms, but the body holds and stores a lot of what we ingest, imbibe, and inhale. Here's a practical way of looking at it: if I eat three meals a day and only use the restroom once that day, where did the other two meals go? If my car needs routine maintenance—oil change, engine flushed, etc.—I must do the same for the living, breathing vehicle known as my body. I'm fully aware that the body has the capability of cleansing itself, but because mine was so severely sick, I had to take measures to help it along until it could get to a place where it was not overloaded.

Amidst all the pain brought on by my healing crisis and the constant anxiety attacks, deep down in the recesses of my soul, there was a knowing that I was under the watchful eye of my Creator. He assured me that this is the road that I must take and that he would personally be there as an unseen guest to guide me. I was being processed, and time and patience would get me through it.

Some days I still felt like I was dying. My spirit felt as if it was leaving my body, and my body felt as if it could not go on anymore. When it got really intense, I cried out to the Father as Yeshua did on the cross, "My God, My God why have you forsaken Me?" (Matthew 27:46 NKJV).

I had to go back to the drawing board. I needed a reprieve, and I had to have it quickly or else I was going to crash and burn. I informed my family that it was imperative for me to fast again.

Lew said, "But you're too weak to fast."

"I know," I responded, "but the foreign matter coming out of me mixed with digested food is causing a binding effect, making it feel as if I am experiencing a traffic jam in my colon." Something had to give. I was miserable. Theodore Roosevelt said, "Courage is not having the strength to go on; it is going on when you don't have the strength."[34] That's what I had to do.

Relying on how fasting made me feel in the past, I decided to take my chance with it, although I was already weak. What did I have to lose? "When you are on a fast 3 days or more, you are really on Mother Nature's and God's miracle operating table. Nature is ridding you of the waste, mucus, toxins, and other foreign substances in your body."[35]

I began a weeklong fast, and it was just what I needed. It unbelievably strengthened my body, mind, and soul. "Hippocrates, Aristotle, Galen, Paracelsus, Plato, Socrates and other great philosophers, scientists, and physicians for centuries have used fasting as a method of cleansing, healing, and renewing the body, mind, and soul."[36] Fasting put everything back into perspective. "Fasting, for example, is a form of self-denial that mimics death. … Death, like pain, strips away the inconsequential."[37]

Lew was concerned about me trying another fast because of the many anxiety attacks and the physical weakness that resulted from my body purging and releasing old matter. Thankfully, I completed my fast with renewed purpose and a brighter outlook on the need to move forward with eating raw food, juices, and smoothies along with incorporating fasting anytime I felt a need to go deeper.

Eating healthy has worked wonders in cleansing my body, but fasting took me even deeper. Eating healthy is like tidying up my house by making sure the clothes are put away, the countertops are pristine, and the floors are swept. Conversely, fasting is like scrubbing the baseboards, getting debris out of the nooks and crannies, and mopping the floors. The level of healing through detoxification and regeneration that I need to experience can only come from the cleansing fire of fasting.

Chapter Nine

Pushing Forward to the Finish Line

**Success is to be measured not so much by the position
that one has reached in life as by the obstacles which one
has overcome while trying to succeed.[38]**
~ Booker T. Washington

In my inbox, something beyond description awaited me. I received another email for a wellness summit. However, this time it was not inviting me to view one; the invitation was for me to participate in one. I was Red Bull pumped and excited.

The invitation was another sign that my persistence in seeking optimal health is paying big dividends. I was given the opportunity to participate in an international documentary titled *The Thyroid Secret*, produced by Dr. Izabella Wentz, PharmD. What an honor! During my interview, I was asked about my diagnosis of Hashimoto Thyroiditis and how it affected my life, my family, and my career. An opportunity to share words of hope with others who were newly diagnosed was also offered. In addition, I was given the distinct honor to thank Dr. Wentz for her contribution in bringing global awareness of thyroid disease, leading to patients receiving an earlier diagnosis.

Seven years have passed since my diagnosis. I have come a long way, and my hope has not waned. I was told by a consultant at Dragon Herbs that for every year I suffered from chronic illness, I would need three months to heal. With that said, seven years have not been enough. Due to the length of time it took to get a diagnosis, I needed another seven years for further healing to be realized. I am not discouraged, though, because I have made remarkable strides. I also made up my mind, midcourse, that I did not want to delay sharing my story or to forfeit any time to encourage others while I wait for my full healing to manifest.

Writing is cathartic for many people, but for me it was a painful reminder of what I did not possess. It is a terrible predicament to desire something so badly and to be on the cusp of achieving it, only to feel as if it slips out of my reach when I attempt to grab it. It is my hope that my experience will jumpstart someone else's health journey. May all my readers reap the benefits of what I have sown in tears, pain, sorrow, and frustration. I had been silenced for years, but God gave me a voice through this book to be a voice for those who have not had a chance to tell their story yet. May you find the wholeness you deserve.

I had to go through the storm to be the lighthouse for someone else. All along, I have been on a direct mission from God, even when my struggle felt like punishment. I often asked God why he had forsaken me, but he hadn't left me. What I went through was training in disguise.

Renovate or Move?

Healing has not been steady; it seems like I take two steps forward and three steps backward. I can sometimes control the process, but I cannot at any time control the outcome. One of the greatest achievements came when the panic attacks stopped. They made me feel as if I had no control over my mind or body. When they occurred, it felt as if I was literally trapped in a tunnel with no oxygen. I felt like I was losing all control of my mind. What a scary and daunting feeling! Thankfully, it's been five years since I had my last panic attack. I'm still on a raw-food diet, eating a variety of fruits, vegetables, nuts, seeds, cold-pressed juices, and smoothies.

My healing crisis, wherein I feel deathly ill due to the endotoxins leaving my body, has been minimal since I have used modalities to cleanse my body at a cellular level, yet masses of obstruction still come out of my body on a daily basis. This is an ongoing testament to how degenerate my body was. One of the major discoveries of deep degeneration is the massive amount of scar tissue my body releases. "The internal scar tissue builds up over the years as a protective life-saving mechanism due to an incorrect lifestyle. This fibrotic scar tissue that your body creates helps to ward off the continual attack of fungus, bad bacteria, viruses and worms that prey on compromised, low integrity, low vibrational tissue."[39]

Out of ignorance, I did not know the foods I was eating were inflammatory, and they were contributing to my health challenges. I have also learned that what I put on my body is important. When I pursued healing, I had to reevaluate cleaning supplies, laundry detergents, my body wash, lotions, hair cremes, lipstick, perfume, and all other body care products. I also had all of my amalgams (silver fillings) removed by a biological dentist and replaced with composite fillings. Everything had to be free of gluten, chemicals, and other harmful ingredients. Once I found out the truth about these harmful items, I stopped using them immediately. I went cold turkey because I wanted to be healed and whole, and I wanted to honor God with my body (the temple) that he has given me and has sustained while I waited for more knowledge to come my way.

I'm reminded of the scripture in the New Covenant which says, "Do you not know that your bodies are temples of the Holy Spirit, who is in you, whom you have received from God? You are not your own; you were bought at a price. Therefore, honor God with your bodies" (1 Corinthians 6:19 NIV).

In my unawareness, the chronic illnesses and the foods I ate created a wasteland in my body. Healing became almost impossible. I shared my temple with viruses, pathogens, creatures, parasites, and other foreign entities that had free range due to what I allowed to be brought into my body through my mouth and various skin products. Those things in and of themselves can sometimes live symbiotically within my body, but when they become overbearing, they can cause considerable damage. Their invasion left my vessel dilapidated and uninhabitable.

I was faced with two choices: to renovate or to move. I chose the daunting, monumental task of renovation. The latter was not even an option since I had a precious daughter to raise, a marriage to sustain, a purpose to fulfill, and a destiny to live out. My family had already lost so much because I physically could not be 100-percent present because of the sickness battles raging within me. It would be premature for them to physically lose me too.

In choosing renovation, I got right down to business. The long, arduous process could only be accomplished in phases. It had taken years to get to this acidic state; therefore, it will take time to heal in reverse. When Lew and I purchased our first home, we had to strip the walls down to the bare studs in order to make it personal to our needs. That's exactly what I have done in order to get the healthy body I desire. All the damage done since I was a child had to be stripped down to the cellular level; I could then start the rebuilding phase. Surface healing was not going to cut it. Many have witnessed the skin healing, the weight loss, and the exceptional glow on my face, but I knew what type of work needed to be done. I had to do the deep inner work no one could see with the naked eye. Although I had outward signs of healing taking place, those signs never truly depicted how deep I needed to go for further healing.

The scar tissue is taking the longest to expel. It did not come out during regular bowel movements. It had to be cleaned out through enemas.

Designed to Heal

My body is masterfully built and equipped with all necessary healing properties already in place. But I have to provide what it needs nutritionally so it can do best what it's designed to do. The astringent fruits like grapefruits, lemons, and grapes had the greatest impact on cleansing and strengthening me internally. "Astringents pull and constrict tissue, pulling toxicity and congestion (mucus) out. At the same time, these foods stimulate the lymphatic and blood flow within the body, allowing the body to get rid of these toxins and mucus."[40]

What I learned is that healing chronic diseases has to be done one day at a time, layer by layer. The wheels of nature turn ever so slowly, yet surely. Think about it. The body is designed to heal. What a liberating thought! I unequivocally understood this because I witnessed it firsthand. Whenever I cut my finger, within days it would be totally healed without any effort on my part.

I've since learned how this principle works when it comes to more serious cases. I knew in my mind that healing was possible. That same knowledge had to be transferred to my heart; now I know it experientially. There's a huge difference in giving mental assent to this truth versus believing and understanding this truth.

I took this truth even further and believed that healing could work also for me. One day, I was thinking extensively about how grateful I am that I survived so many years with chronic diseases running rampant in my body. Every time I went to my massage therapist, she asked, "Have you ever thought to thank your body for helping you to stay alive after all you have been through?" My answer was always a resounding "no" because my first thought of gratitude was not to my body but to my Creator. I do not ever want to put the creation above the Creator.

The very thought that I am still on this earth, in retrospect, makes me feel so special. I know that I am a medical anomaly. When I tell my story to others, they too are astonished. Strangers whom I've met along the way have asked me for my name so they can be on the lookout for more information about how I overcame such dire circumstances.

Besides my personal healing, I know that the reason I am still alive is to be an encouragement to others. My pain must have purpose. My test was producing a testimony. My mess must involve a message. Otherwise, why else would I still be here? I'm not still alive just to say I exist, but I've seen that there's a divine purpose for me to be here. I must share my story and help others live their lives to the fullest. Willpower alone emphatically cannot sustain the type of trauma and heartache I endured. Divine purpose is what sustained me then and sustains me now.

Letter to My Body

With those thoughts coursing through my mind, I was firmly impressed to write a letter to my body thanking her for upholding me during all I had gone through. I was excited to write this letter as a means to honor my body, but I had no clue how to start it or end it. The first thing that I did was open up the Notes app on my iPad, then I just started typing. To my amazement, the words began to flow. My fingers did not quit typing until the letter was completed. What I had written shocked me.

Dear body,

First and foremost, I want to thank you for all that you have done for me. Beyond a shadow of a doubt, you have been my most loyal friend. From birth, you have stuck with me and fought for me. You are the only reason that I'm privileged to live life on this planet called Earth. Your unique mode of transportation allows me to go from place to place at will. It is through you that I get to experience all that this life has to offer. From your coffers, to name a few, I am acquainted with love, happiness, joy, peace, sadness, disappointments, sickness, and health. All are experienced through you in this life.

For years, you attempted to directly communicate with me concerning unforeseen trouble and the many pitfalls that could occur should I disregard your promptings, but I was conditioned to ignore your subtle warnings. When I was nudged by you to express out loud some of my symptoms, others told me that they oftentimes experienced the same thing; therefore unitedly those traits were deemed as normal.

Through divine persuasion, you spoke louder and clearer. Thankfully, I listened to you. I longed to make right what I had done to you, but honestly, I was at a loss of where I should start. You have been poked, pricked, cut, aspirated, smashed, and x-rayed in an all-out attempt to find out how to silence your screams. No viable answer was ever given. Each doctor's visit confirmed your desperate plea. I often wondered, how could I possibly fix all the systems that were beginning to break down and degenerate? Each passing day, week, month, and year, your symptoms grew increasingly worse, yet trying to get assistance that you desperately craved seemed nearly impossible. I, too, diligently searched for someone to help, but no one ever came. Thankfully, I was awakened by the light of divine love before I utterly destroyed you. King Solomon, the wisest man that ever lived, said, "The spirit of a man can endure his sickness, but who can survive a broken spirit?" (Proverbs 18:14 BSB). My spirit was broken from all the pain that I caused you.

One day, after years of pleading and begging for assistance, you were told by a man wearing a white coat and an apparatus around his neck that you have an autoimmune disease. A few short months later, another team discovered three more of these diseases. What was I thinking? I should have known that this was not the beginning or ending of our entire story. I know you far better than anyone else on this planet. You would never attack me or betray me. Despite what it looked like and the ugly names that you were called, you were doing everything you possibly could to keep me alive until divine intervention could get me into a posture that I could hear beyond my natural ears. All the while you held firmly to your mandate that you are fearfully and wonderfully made. The One who formed you spoke these words into your DNA, and you were unshaken in your resolve. When no one else would listen, you stayed true to our Creator, and you did everything in your power to cover me. You are the true Ride or Die, the real MVP, the GOAT.

One day, I heard the three most glorious words that changed the trajectory of my very existence in this realm called life. These combined words are not new, but they caused a radical shift in me. When I heard them, they were reminiscent of what we heard our Creator speak. When these words fell gently on your ears, the reverberation sent an electrical current throughout your body and into my spirit. At that moment, new life sprang forth just like in the beginning of time. Darkness dissipated, and hope sprang into action. The plan to regenerate you began to unfold daily. The three words—"You can heal!"—carried such miraculous efficacy that the magnitude of their meaning was incomprehensible. I recall how you leapt with excitement upon hearing these words. In times past, these words were elusive. But now was the appointed time. Small but mighty, they replaced all the negative words I had ever heard about you. These three words took up residence in me and immediately began to clean out the old to make room for their all-encompassing power. They begin to slough off obstruction like icicles melting on a warm sunny day.

Each waking hour, I position myself to receive the downloads that *Elohim*, the creator God, graciously gives to me. He soundlessly imparts exactly what is needed, and I follow his instructions with what a former pastor called "scrupulous exactitude." Cooperating with this original design of vibrant health has not been a walk in the park. Coming into alignment and agreement will be the key to unlock new potential. You are doing what you are designed to do, and I am cooperating by removing all things that caused you to function in a less than optimal fashion. Together, in harmony, we will experience the joy and bliss of health, which was intended from the very beginning of creation, unencumbered by sickness and disease. When the renovation is complete, my life on earth will take on new meaning. The level of suffering that we shared will be no more. Together, we will collectively bring the plan of eternity to the earthly realm.

Body, please accept my sincerest apologies, and thank you again for working hard for me as we recover all that was lost.

Yours truly,
Dawn G. Green

A Hydro Colon Therapist

Although there was now full cooperation between us—mind, body, and spirit—many times I wondered why the masses got lodged in my colon and caused so much pain, not only in my lower region but throughout my entire body. I recall one summer my journal entry read "God, please tell me what's inside my body that's wreaking so much havoc, and tell me how do I get it out." The pain was so severe that oftentimes I could not physically put one foot in front of the other in order to walk from point A to point B.

That prayer prompted me to search further for help. Each step of the way, I had to go through a new process; there were no quick fixes. To find some semblance of relief, I added a hydro colon therapist to my team. The cleansing of my body was happening so rapidly I could not keep up with it through enemas alone.

Before my first appointment, I met with the owner to inquire if her colonic machine could handle the amount of cellular waste that was passing through my colon. She chuckled. Unbeknownst to her, she was about to witness something she had never seen.

During my first colon hydrotherapy session, an enormous amount of mucus, scar tissue, crystallized stones, and cellular waste was released. It was obvious that sickness ran deep into the cellular level of my tissues and organs. Many layers had to be peeled back. The amount of waste that was dispelled called for an unusual number of colonics in a short period of time. Around my fiftieth session, the water was pitch black. I continued to return because seeing the changes during those sessions were proof positive that my body was going through this wonderful metamorphosis. Each session the therapist pumped water through my colon, and when she released the water, the amount of waste was astonishing. Most people get colonics seasonally. In my case, I had to schedule one every week. Depending on how much matter I was releasing, she might suggest a second one that same week.

Repeated colonic irrigations, where approximately eight gallons of water is pumped into my colon to flush out its contents, still weren't sufficient. When I got home, I often gave myself an enema. This was due to the fact that foreign matter was being released so quickly from my body that I couldn't empty my colon fast enough. My body's cleansing process was extremely powerful, and I wanted to help facilitate it with everything that I could do.

Within two years, I had over seventy-five colonics, costing me thousands of dollars. Looking back, it was well worth the investment. I'm grateful for financial and health reasons that I don't have to have as many sessions anymore. I am on a yearly schedule now versus a weekly one.

A Loving, Caring Husband

Because I was unable to work outside of the home, all the financial responsibility has fallen on Lew's shoulders. He has taken care of me for over thirty-two years of marriage. I silently watched as my sickness had an unfavorable effect on him. He worries greatly about me. He has sacrificed hundreds of thousands of dollars trying to get medical help for me. He was the one who held me at night when I was hurting. Many people empathize with the one that is sick, but they sometimes forget the struggles of the caregiver. Lew goes above and beyond to see that we have everything we need. Even though he loves and enjoys taking care of and providing for his family, the weight of it all is evident from the puffiness under his eyes and the rapidly graying of his hair. Despite it all, he maintains a happy disposition, but his countenance looks weary. When I look into his green eyes, I see a reflection of myself; his eyes are filled with questions and a deep longing for answers. He wants to know when the reward will outweigh the effort as much as I do.

Lew has been a loving, caring friend since my early twenties. He willingly married me with full knowledge of my health challenges. When he asked me to be his wife, I sat with him and told him all about my physical challenges before I said, "Yes." I couldn't withhold this information from him. He deserved full disclosure. In the final analysis, I wanted a relationship based on truth, honesty, and integrity. Therefore, I made sure I told him everything. Given these points, the decision to marry me rested solely on him. When I asked him if he still wanted to marry me after hearing my story, he said, "Yes."

With Lew's affirmative agreement to become one with a young woman whose body was so broken, I was emboldened to ask God for a new body. I was taught from my youth that at the resurrection I will be given a new body to live in throughout eternity, but I wanted a new one on earth so I could enjoy a long life and carry out my purpose.

I had no way of knowing how that obscure prayer would be answered or that the bounty for its manifestation would come with a hefty price. I had no idea that the fight for my health would mean coming face-to-face with death. If I had known the full scope, I may not have embarked on this path.

Born Again

Thankfully, God does not give us all the details when we decide to do something significant. I thought the hardest part was to go from a 100-percent organic diet to a fully raw one, sacrificing all the foods I love and enjoy. I thought giving up my traditional Thanksgiving, birthday, anniversary, and every other holiday meal would be sacrificial. But when these events came and went, I was fine.

I should have known that opposition of the worst kind was waiting for me. Nothing monumental ever comes easy, and it is worth the fight. It cost me physically, emotionally, financially, relationally, and spiritually. I found myself in the dark, deep place of the abyss. But I kept pushing and fighting against the chains that tried to hold me back from escaping their grip. I cried out for help relentlessly. Taking back my health from the unforeseen forces was no easy feat. That stronghold did not want to give up its place of habitation that it had grown accustomed to for many decades. I had to "accept the challenge so that I can feel the exhilaration of victory."[41]

There have been small victories along the way, amidst the grueling days. But I must continue to push forward to the finish line. In order to fully heal, I had to understand the law of thrust. Sickness tried to hold me back and keep me where I was, but I had to break through that barrier and overcome. Like Chuck Yeager, who broke the sound barrier, I must thrust forward until I achieve optimal health. The test of time is not as important as the certainty of victory.

With the desire of a new body lingering in the distance, I vividly remember a dream that I had before I got the diagnosis. In my dream, I was in, I presume, my mother's womb ready to be born. I can feel my mom's body pulsating with contractions, which were crucial in gently pushing me up the birth canal through her pelvic bones. I recall that with each contraction, I was able to move up a little further; when the contractions stopped, I stopped. As I continued through the birth canal, I felt every movement. It was rhythmic. When my head came through the vaginal opening, I saw and felt two blue latex-gloved hands help pull me out the rest of the way into this new world. When I awoke from my dream, I proclaimed, "I'm being born again." This birthing was a sign that I would be given a fresh start to right my wrongs and begin my life again, healed and symptom free.

Chapter Ten

Lighting a Path for Others

**One day you will tell your story of how you overcame
what you went through [in your darkest moments,] and
it will become someone else's survival guide.**[42]

~ Brene Brown

On my road to healing, I have had some tremendous
successes. I have watched my health rejuvenate in ways I
had only dreamed about. My long-haul symptoms began
to diminish. There have been no other cysts. The severe
pains in my stomach subsided due to removing gluten and other
inflammatory foods that did not agree with my physical makeup,
then allowing my gut time to heal. My lab work is starting to show
promising signs that I'm on the mend. Excitedly, I watched my
skin clear up and various rashes I had incurred over the years
instantly disappear. Moles and other skin tags miraculously
vanished. I have not had any more fainting spells; my never-ending
headaches have ceased; my heart palpitations are completely gone.
My recurring ear infection no longer exists, and as a bonus, I have
lost a considerable amount of weight.

I am extremely grateful for these astronomical strides, yet I
am still working through some detours, so I have to reevaluate
where I am today compared to where I was seven years ago. The
work behind me was considerable, but there is more work to be
done. Today, autoimmune has come in and out of remission; yet I
refuse to give up on the person I could be; neither will I say
goodbye to the person I want to become. Remission is not out of
my reach. I will continue until I discover that missing puzzle piece
that will complete the plan I have already instituted. Like it did
years ago, my intuition has once again kicked in, and I believe the

answer to optimal health lies in my gut—in the deep crevices of my intricate microbiome.

Triggers and Stressors

As in construction projects, when it is time to renovate, you never know what lies ahead until you start the demolition process. I personally feel as if I am stumbling out from the ruins of a collapsed building. As I changed my diet and began to eat highly alkaline foods that were astringent in nature, those foods, along with proteolytic enzymes, began to break down the hard debris inside me on the cellular level. Once those layers were chipped away, my body began to respond favorably.

With chronic illnesses, anything external or internal can trigger and upset your body's ecosystem. Environment, food, stress, trauma, nutritional deficiencies, lack of sleep—the list goes on. Recently, I've encountered stress in ways I never experienced before. A myriad of circumstances caused my body to respond once more in a fight-or-flight modality. I became worried beyond measure when Mikayla, in her first year of college, went through a major adjustment period of finding her way socially, mentally, and physically. She endured excessive sickness, going in and out of the hospital, all while being away from home.

Other stressors occurred when I once again needed to look for specific medical help for things happening within my body. In our search, Lew and I traveled long distances to find a holistic, experienced doctor to work with my specific need, but to no avail. Although I have made drastic dietary changes and I am very careful about what products I use on my skin, hair, and body, I have surprisingly become extremely sensitive to certain foods, herbs, and medications. What I was able to tolerate prior to the overhaul of my diet, my body can no longer handle. These new occurrences signaled to me that the issue may be related to my gut health and the state of my microbiome. But as of yet, I haven't had any doctor medically confirm that.

I noticed the subtle changes, and then they quickly escalated. I shared with Lew the importance of finding a doctor who understands chronic illnesses and their nuances, along with how to heal and restore the gut. The doctor must be very knowledgeable in all these areas so he can use his expertise to guide and treat me holistically with as little stress to me as possible. Yes, stress is definitely highest on the list for my number one trigger. I'm working diligently to manage it as best as I can.

With all the work I have done thus far, my physical challenges have depleted me and robbed me of the ability to bring as much benefit to my family as I thought I would be able to by now. Oftentimes, I am left feeling devalued in a world that over-emphasizes production. I simply cannot do what I used to be able to do. I have the desire but not the strength.

At this juncture, I was hoping to be gainfully employed and to be more spontaneous with family outings and vacations. To date, everything I do is still so methodical. It's almost impossible to just get up and go like I once did. Even when we are traveling locally around town, I have to pack my food so we do not have to stop and purchase from places that may not cater to my specific dietary restrictions. Planning a trip via a plane is monumental because extensive research has to be done prior to reaching my destination to ensure that the area I am traveling to will have a variety of food I can eat to sustain me for whatever length of time I will be there. Traveling long distance by car has been the best option for me because I can bring everything I could possibly need with me. The only downfall is that road trips are entirely too long. I usually pack everything in my kitchen I can think of "except the kitchen sink."

The Good within Reach

I'm learning all over again how to care for myself in new, exciting ways. My body continues to purge the old waste matter that had become cemented to my organs, tissues, and cells. Healing at this magnitude sometimes leaves me questioning my wisdom, sanity, and approach. Healing looks different depending upon my physical or mental state. Oftentimes this fluctuation has brought me seismic uncertainty. Chronic illness was my body's way of letting me know it desperately needed help. Once I knew better, I heeded the call, and I will stay the course until my goal is achieved. Navy SEAL

Eric Greitens says, "Resilience is the virtue that enables people to move through hardship and become better. No one escapes pain, fear, and suffering. Yet from pain can come wisdom, from fear can come courage, from suffering can come strength."[43] I must continue to be resilient.

Author Jonas Salzgeber writes, "No tree becomes deep-rooted and sturdy unless strong winds blow against it. This shaking and pulling is what makes the tree tighten its grip and plant its roots more securely."[44] Like a mighty oak that can weather any storm, I must stay strong. Constant physical pain makes daily-life enjoyment fleeting. I'm not in pain from the food I'm eating; I'm in pain from the effects of autoimmune disease that is still trying to leave my body. Life with invisible illnesses (they are called invisible illnesses because you don't outwardly look sick) has been extremely hard, but life keeps whispering its promises to me, encouraging me to continue my fight until the end.

Anyone can rejoice and be happy when life is going well. One may even find hope when confronted with a problem here or there. But relentless health challenges coupled with financial hardship can make you question your efforts. For a long time, I had no one with whom to share intimate, insecure feelings that bombarded my soul. For every pain I encountered, I wished I had had someone to help me navigate through it. Would I know the joy and bliss of being well? That question plagued me for years. The promises that life keeps whispering to me … only time will prove her right.

Just like my illnesses are invisible, so are my sadness and fears. It wasn't that I pretended to be happy when I was sad; in fact, I've learned to compartmentalize my feelings and emotions. I only share with those with whom I feel safe. I must know unequivocally that whomever I open up with will take the knowledge that I share and treat it as if it's his or her most prized possession. "Aside from the challenges of facing each day, one of the most difficult and often hurtful consequences is the lack of understanding from others … we are trying to deal with a condition(s) that leaves us feeling drained, mentally and physically."[45]

Despite it all, I have learned to carry on and face my giants and bring each one down to its knees so I can disarm it and eventually annihilate all of them in pursuit of my victory. We are called to hard places. Faith is a muscle, and it must be tested. These painstaking times awakened me to the good that was in reach all along.

The Aftermath of Long-Term Disease

At the onset, my determination to fight seemed unmatched to that of my opponent. Yet a force higher than me propelled me onward. Although my darkest hours were always so relentless, I girded up my loins and stood guard over my mind like a heavily armed soldier. I used the Holy Scriptures as ammunition to annihilate the enemy trying to destroy me. I constantly checked my spiritual armor to be sure that it was sealed up at every entry point (see Ephesians 6:10–17). I knew that if I let up for even a moment, that would be the end of me. I stood firm in my resolve. There was no wiggle room to relax. The warfare was too intense. For certain, my character has been forged in the fire of adversity as it was bombarded with unrelenting blows and assaults. My breath was constantly being snatched from me. The moment I found a semblance of hope, tragedy struck again.

One devasting blow happened in my sixth year of recovery. After I had spent all those years fully changing my diet and embracing a healthier lifestyle, I lost the use of my right arm for several weeks. After the second week of it not getting better, I decided to go to a medical acupuncturist to see if acupuncture could restore its use. I am an independent woman, and having my husband bathe and dress me was not a good feeling. The doctor said that inflammation was the culprit for the nonuse of my arm. In addition to acupuncture, she gave me herbs to take to quiet the inflammation.

Months after that, following a good night sleep, I awakened to discover that I could not walk. The inability to walk lasted for approximately two weeks. Not knowing what to do because I hadn't done anything to cause this to happen, I just waited and let it resolve itself.

Shortly after that, I experienced excruciating pain in a lower tooth that seemed to come out of nowhere. I could not eat at all due to the pain. In order to prevent malnourishment, I did a lot of juicing and drank smoothies. I chose liquids that were nutritionally dense while I gave my tooth time to heal. None of these occurrences made sense to me, but I'm fully aware they are the aftermath of long-term disease.

Supernatural Grace

It is my hope that the difficulties of my circumstances and the stamina to persevere will light a path for others. We have more knowledge and more access to knowledge today than this world has ever experienced. In addition to utilizing all the knowledge available, I have chosen to cling to the Life-giver that I've put my hope in. Nothing in this life satisfies the longing of my soul except God.

When others learn about all the catastrophes I've encountered, they may marvel at how I am still standing. For me, I've placed the whole of myself into the secret place of God's love. I have never been abandoned, although at times it appeared as if I was. When I look back over my journey, the times when it seemed as if I was walking alone, it was not my footsteps I was seeing but the footsteps of the One who carried me.

Seven years ago, when I first got diagnosed, everything about life looked different. The world today is not the same. With everything going on in me, around me, and in the world, I had to put guardrails around my heart so I would not fall off the precipice into despair.

I fully understand that the moment we were born, we began the passage of quietly and slowly dying. With me, I felt death in my body continuously. Every health battle I fought consistently required extraordinary exertion and formidable strength to triumph over the unforeseen forces that seemed to overwhelm me. The warm covering of grace that shielded me all these years and which allowed me to go through each fiery trial like a champ seemed to have been momentarily stripped away, leaving me vulnerable and depleted.

Hindsight has proven that it wasn't my strong will to live nor my determined personality alone that kept me thriving. It was supernatural grace. For whatever reason, whenever grace seemed to take wings and fly away from me, a cold chill of fright ravaged my soul. Even in the confines of my warm house, I could literally feel brisk, frigid air blow through me as if I were naked. "What is happening now?" I asked. "How did I get to this place? I feel as if I'm stuck on the highway of healing. I need to get off at the next exit and get on the street called 'Healed.'"

There were days, weeks, and months on end that I was extremely exhausted—the kind of exhaustion no amount of sleep or nutrition could resolve. I felt as if someone had beaten me mercilessly, dragged me for miles and miles, then left me for dead. I tried everything I could to get the proper rest that would lead to cell regeneration and renewal. I often asked myself, "How do I disassociate from it all in order to rest from sickness?" It was always present. No getting away from it.

I learned that rest came with persistence. In the midst of tiredness, I had to persevere until my body caught up with all the nutrition, rest, nurture, and protocols I was daily administering. I cannot reiterate enough … true health takes time, especially when you are reversing a lifetime of disease.

As the healing journey progressed, there were times when my lifeline seemed quiet. The little signs in the beginning that showed I was on the right road slowly faded into the distance, especially when the journey got unbearably tough. Each little breakthrough meant everything to me. It was like a ray of sunshine that burst forth as I basked in the warm embrace of my heavenly Father's love. In looking back over these seven years, I realize that the omnipotent Divine Presence carried me through my most difficult times.

Through it all, I mastered the art of showing up as my best self. By nature, I'm not a complainer. I'm a fixer. I'm told that people love being around me because I have a God-given ability to lift heavy hearts even when I can't lift my own heart. I always find a reason to smile.

For seven years, I consistently worked for change. The change I longed for was called "healed" not "remission." At this point, I'm not settling, but I will take what I can get. As racecar driver Bobby Unser said, "Success is where preparation and opportunity meet."[46] I will be here and present and available when healing arrives.

Expecting to Win

Year after year, I have sat on a metal chair with a mesh covering on my deck at the back of my house and watched the seasons come and go—summer, fall, winter, spring. I am fascinated by the mysterious ways the acorns randomly fall from the tree so the squirrels below its branches can gather and store up food for the winter ahead. Without fail, I have witnessed the leaves change from several hues of green into a myriad of vibrant colors. Within a short time, those colorful leaves softly pull themselves away from their branches, leaving the full and bountiful tree bare.

Change proved to be inevitable—each season in its unique order. As I meticulously studied nature on my back deck, I often wondered when my body would heed the order of shedding, healing, and regeneration that was inscribed in its DNA long before creation took its course. Everything in nature informs me of the disorder that inhabits me, which brought me to the place of pain that I must carefully and methodically unravel so I can loosen the grip of disease that will allow my body to enjoy the full benefit associated with change.

Strangely, as I get closer to my victory, the intensity of the battle thickens. What's different from this fight today than the fight from seven years ago? I'm expecting to win versus just surviving. Each layer that is peeled away from my body brings a new set of challenges. Each waking moment, I must connect with my command center, my heavenly Father, to obtain wisdom and knowledge for each new set of circumstances.

I've never fought a battle this intense and detailed. The unknowing boggles my mind, the hardness of the struggle seems to weaken my body, and the lengthiness of the battle assails my spirit. Each day all three—mind, body, spirit—have to be strengthened, fortified, and ministered to in order for me to have the wherewithal to rise and do it all over again the next day.

To obtain optimal health, I had to use the same brute force in which the velocity of the disease was delivered to me. I had to match force with force. I'm finally waking up to what has always been. Many viewed my sickness as "oh, she's just sick," but my sickness was a halting of life, a cessation of vibrancy, a wrenching of my soul, a stagnation of my full potential, a life lost in the cacophony of all the devastation that sickness and disease bring.

When people close to you cannot see or understand your grind, they dismiss you as lazy, unmotivated, and lacking a viable plan. What they don't know is that when you are reversing a number of chronic diseases, you have zero time to invest in anything that looks like it will bring you visible success but will actually take you away from the hidden and most important task at hand if you indulge in it.

The Possibility of Wholeness

True healing is not glamorous. It is not on display and deemed desirable. Each day my heart flutters for fear of running out of time. The twenty-four hours in my day are filled with researching, praying, and listening for strategies to restore my body to a place it has never seen. Whatever time remains, I use to implement the strategies I've learned. Where is there room for anything else? No one can answer that question unless they have walked in my shoes.

Other people will never understand my journey. It is mine alone. I do not even expect anyone to remotely understand. All I ask for are kindness and compassion. Words should be crafted to heal and not to hurt. Some of the things people have said to me were well-meaning but callous: "You don't look sick," and "Well, you're still here," and "Have you tried this supplement, yoga, meditation, speaking the Word?" Or they asked, "Why can't you eat that food?" and "When are you going to do this and that?" Those questions and comments seemed dismissive and heartless.

One of the best things anybody can say to one who is chronically ill is "How can I support you?" My hope for getting well was escalated because I wanted to eradicate and extinguish those types of questions. Comments like those hurt down to the soul. Maybe they would not cause so much pain in normal circumstances, but they do hurt those who are chronically ill because the pain of illness runs so deeply.

I've become fully aware of the process needed to heal. My hope is that many more will come to that realization. Mine came later than I expected, but thankfully, the tools necessary to heal have been afforded to me and the awareness of other healing modalities are rapidly peeking over the horizon. The delay of healing nearly killed me. I was constantly gasping for breath. I wanted to live the most vibrant life ever, but life seemed to mock me.

When the time had come and I was all in and ready for this great, wonderful change, I was strategically placed on God's operating table. He metaphorically took his heavenly electrode paddles and applied them to my flatlined and hopeless heart. I was jolted to an awakening that I had never known before. That awakening was the beginning of the countless trials that I had to endure to see the results I longed for. I'm reminded of the man in the New Covenant who was sick for thirty-eight years at the pool of Bethesda (see John 5:1–6). The first question Yeshua asked him was "Do you want to be made well?" He had to ask the man that question due to the length of his illness and the difficulty of getting well. Someone had to ignite the spark of hope in him, the possibility of being made whole.

God Is Ever Present

This healing journey is not for the faint of heart. When I decided to get on the path of cellular healing, I intrinsically lost all control of my life and its outcomes. Disappointment drew me deeper into the arms of my Creator. The shallowness of this world became my driving force to know that God's Word is true, and I so desperately needed it to jump off the pages and be a reality in my life. When I set my mind to follow the plan that he laid out for me, the road was bumpy and long. Many days it felt as if God gave me a directive and then went to a distant land, leaving me alone to figure things out on my own. Each day I called out to him, but my cry seemed to fall on deaf ears. He felt too far away.

The hardest part for me was when my prayers seemed impenetrable. I was delirious with disappointment. During my desperation, I could literally feel an iron barrier between my prayers and his heart. In my humanity I often said, "God, you have the power to help me change my circumstances, so why do you refuse? Why would you allow me to continue to suffer when I'm calling out to you for help?"

My journal proves that, at times, I questioned his timing and his refusal to come to my aid. His lack of response was hurtful, yet I continued to rehearse his words, even when they seemed powerless and left me emotionally wounded and afraid. That's the paradox of being a spiritual being living in a human body. I wanted so desperately to trust him with all of my heart, but his apparent abandonment made me terribly frightened.

I know that people will not always be there for you, but I take joy in knowing that God is ever present. What I want is all that I can conceive. but with a vast God there is so much more than meets the eye. Nothing makes sense when you are in the throes of it. Hindsight is always 20/20. Thankfully, time answers and reveals all things.

The struggle and his non-responsiveness were designed for my growth and dependency upon him, even when I could not sense his presence. I knew that his covenant proved that he loved me. Therefore, I had to blindly trust that his love story for me had not been rewritten and that it remained just like he said it would. My journey to health was filled with changing scenarios and plot twists. That's when supernatural faith kicked into gear.

All faith must be tested. Living between what was and what I long for has brought much disappointment. Although I seemed disillusioned, there was an ever-present, unseen force drawing me to the One my heart longed for. I had to painstakingly bury the thought of what I perceived healing looked like and just allow healing to unfold without stressing over it. My body ached to get back to the state of its original design. As sickness permeated my body, it lamented with anguish and pain to return to the place etched in my DNA.

Life on the road to healing was such a roller coaster. Healing is not in a straight line. Healing is messy at times. On days when I thought I had it all together and started to soar above the clouds, in an instant, it was as if someone reached up and snatched me right out of the place where I started to see things from an aerial perspective. The pain of all that I had endured came rushing back in to mock me as if I had never started this journey.

All of this time, I thought I was a misfit, yet in reality, I was chosen. I was handpicked to go through this suffering so I would be stronger to help others and to be the voice for those who, for whatever reason, cannot tell their story yet.

Passionately Pursuing Optimal Health

True regenerative healing is painful. It comes at a cost. But once I put my hand to the plough to break up the fallow ground, I could not go back (see Luke 9:62). On many days I wrestled with what was and what I was hoping for. What was and what I hoped for fought tooth and nail, like gangbangers trying to take territory. At times the answer of hope seemed light years away, but the divine in me would not let me give up optimism, despite how I felt. It was difficult to enjoy life to its fullest, mainly because the hard task of undoing years of being unhealthy demanded most of my waking hours.

Healing for me was all consuming. Inwardly, I was running at a breakneck speed in my endeavor to accomplish all my tasks before the day's end so I could eke out time to spend quality moments with Lew and Mikayla. More often than not, my plans fell to the ground, and I was left disappointed and broken. Sickness robbed me of decades of family time. Therefore, I desperately wanted and needed those times to be redeemed. I often prayed, "Lord, restore to me the years that the cankerworm, the palmerworm, the locust, and [Dawn] have eaten" (see Joel 2:25). I included myself because I'm not exempt from my responsibility.

Short of a miracle, returning to wholeness takes time. I had to divide my love affair with obtaining optimal health with the loves of my life, Lew and Mikayla. It's hard to painlessly parent when you are devoid of strength. On rare occasions, I was actually happy that they were out of the house for a few hours so I could focus wholeheartedly on what my body needed to do to heal without the pressure that they too needed my attention.

When my body was doing its heaviest detoxing, I felt even more sick. As the old, embedded obstruction continued to slough off, the residue traveled through my blood stream, and it felt as if someone had poisoned me. Until it was expelled, I felt weak and constantly on the verge of nausea. Some of the healing modalities and protocols I use to help me combat the more intense healing crises are infrared saunas, jumping on my trampoline, a whole body vibration plate, dry brushing, Pulsed Electromagnetic Field Therapy (PEFDT), ear candling, Epsom salts baths, and sipping lots of adaptogenic Tulsi Holy Basil Tea.

While I wait for my healing dreams to come true and to live the life of health I'm destined for, I continue to do my part. I will emphatically continue to employ perseverance, patience, and hope. Despite the length of time that it took to get a diagnosis and all the pain and suffering I have endured, I realize that I am in the exact place I prayed for—it just doesn't look like what I imagined healing to be. No way is this the beginning or ending of my story but a continuation as I passionately pursue optimal health.

I unequivocally know that the body is designed to heal. May you gain the tools needed to be your own health advocate. You too can heal. It is my greatest hope that you can muster the courage to learn and explore your unique body, to discover what works best for you, and to use the tools I have shared so you also can take charge of your well-being and overcome obstacles for optimal health. Let us collectively be the lighthouse to shine the light of healing so that with one voice, we all can tell our story.

Endnotes

[1] "Me and you, us never part," *The Color Purple*, directed by Steven Spielberg (1985; Burbank, CA: Warner Home Video, 1997), DVD.

[2] "Tori Amos," TreasureQuotes, accessed July 25, 2023, https://www.treasurequotes.com/quotes/healing-takes-courage-and-we-all-have-courage.

[3] "Dolly Parton Quotes," GoodReads, accessed July 25, 2023, https://www.goodreads.com/quotes/347761-we-cannot-direct-the-wind-but-we-can-adjust-the.

[4] "Maya Angelou, Quotes," Goodreads, accessed July 6, 2023, https://www.goodreads.com/quotes/335-when-someone-shows-you-who-they-are-believe-them-the.

[5] "Lucius Annaeus Seneca Quotes," BrainyQuote, accessed July 25, 2023, https://www.brainyquote.com/quotes/lucius_annaeus_seneca_163843.

[6] Debi Walker, N.D.,"Breast Thermography: History, Theory, and Use: Is this screening tool adequate for standalone use?" Natural Medicine Journal, February 11, 2014, https://www.naturalmedicinejournal.com/journal/breast-thermography-history-theory-and-use.

[7] "Hippocrates Quotes," AZQuotes, accessed July 25, 2023, https://www.azquotes.com/author/22138-Hippocrates.

[8] Xiaoping Liu, Xio Change, Siyand Leng, et al., "Detection for Disease Tipping Points by Landscape Dynamic Network Biomarkers," *National Science Review* 6:4 (July 2019), 775–785, published online December 28, 2018, https://academic.oup.com/nsr/article/6/4/775/5266397?login=false.

[9] "Amenorrhea," Mayo Clinic, accessed February 20, 2020, https://www.mayoclinic.org/diseases-conditions/amenorrhea/symptoms-causes/syc-20369299.

[10] "Insanity Is Doing the Same Thing Over and Over Again and Expecting Different Results," QuoteInvestigator, March 23, 2017, https://quoteinvestigator.com/2017/03/23/same/.

[11] "Non-Alcoholic Fatty Liver Disease, NAFLD," American Liver Foundation, accessed February 21, 2020, https://liverfoundation.org/liver-diseases/fatty-liver-disease/nonalcoholic-fatty-liver-disease-nafld/.

[12] "About Epstein-Barr Virus EBV," Center for Disease Control and Prevention, accessed February 21, 2020, www.cdc.gov/epstein-barr/about-ebv.html.

[13] "What Oprah Knows for Sure about Real Power," Oprah.com, accessed July 24, 2023, https://www.oprah.com/spirit/what-oprah-knows-for-sure-about-real-power.

[14] Amy McKenna, "15 Nelson Mandela Quotes," Britannica, accessed July 10, 2023, https://www.britannica.com/list/nelson-mandela-quotes.

[15] "Barbara Kingsolver Quotes," Goodreads, accessed July 12, 2023, https://www.goodreads.com/quotes/363583-the-very-least-you-can-do-in-your-life-is.

[16] "Zig Ziglar Quotes," BrainyQuote, accessed July 25, https://www.brainyquote.com/quotes/zig_ziglar_617848.

[17] Saul Mcleod, PhD, "Maslow's Hierarchy of Needs," Simple Psychology, updated on July 26, 2023, https://www.simplypsychology.org/maslow.html.

[18] Allan Wechsler, "Keeping the Shabbos: Orthodox in an Un-orthodox World," Chabad.org, accessed February 22, 2020, https://www.chabad.org/library/article_cdo/aid/93788/jewish/keepinmg-the-Shabbos.htm.

[19] "Shabbos: The Real Existence," SimpleToRemember.com, accessed February 26, 2020, (excerpt from *Living Inspired* by Rabbi D Akiva Tatz), https://www.simpletoremember.com/articles/a/shabbos-shabbat/.

[20] "Shabbos: The Real Existence."

[21] "Maimonides Quotes," Goodreads, accessed July 25, 2023, https://www.goodreads.com/quotes/379141-no-disease-that-can-be-treated-by-diet-should-be.

[22] T. D. Jakes, Foreword to *Lost and Found: Finding Hope in the Detours of Life* by Sarah Jakes, Reprint edition, (Grand Rapids, MI: Bethany House Publishers, 2015) 9.

[23] Dr. Izabella Wentz, PharmMD, "Recommended Labs," ThyroidPharmacist, accessed July 25, 2023. https://thyroidpharmacist.com/recommended-labs.

[24] "Betrayal: The Autoimmune Disease Solution They're Not Telling You," Docuseries by Dr. Tom O'Bryan, thedr.com, accessed April 2023, https://thedr.com/autoimmune-solution.

[25] "Fasting Quotes," AllAboutFasting.com, accessed July 17, 2023, https://www.allaboutfasting.com/fasting-quotes.html.

[26] Paul C. Bragg and Patricia Bragg, "The Miracle of Fasting: Proven throughout History for Physical, Mental, & Spiritual Rejuvenation," 2004. PDF File.

[27] Robert Morse, N.D., *The Detox Miracle Sourcebook: Raw Foods and Herbs for Complete Cellular Regeneration,* e-book edition, (London: One World Press, 2012) 104.

[28] Morse, *The Detox Miracle Sourcebook,* 104.

[29] "Christine Caine Quotes," QuoteFancy, accessed July 17, 2023, https://quotefancy.com/quote/1702887/Christine-Caine-The-pain-of-recovery-is-sometimes-worse-than-the-pain-of-the-injury-Allow.

[30] Andree-Anne Boisvert, Matthew P. Chang, Don C. Sheppard, et al., "Microbial Biofilms in Pulmonary and Critical Care Diseases," NIH: National Library of Medicine, First published in *Annals of the American Thoracic Society*, 13:9 (2016): 1615–23, https://pubmed.ncbi.nlm.nih.gov/27348071/.

[31] Darrell Wolfe, Dr., *Healthy to 100: The Ultimate Guide to Bullet Proofing Your Body Against Disease, Eliminating Pain, Burning Fat and Living Longer*, E-book edition, (Wolfe Publishing, 2016), 97.

[32] Izabella Wentz, PharmD, FASCP, "The 5 Stages of Hashimoto's Thyroiditis," ThryoidPharmicist, accessed August 14, 2022, https://thyroidpharmacist.com/articles/5-stages-hashimotos-thyroiditis/.

[33] St. John of the Cross, "The Dark Night of the Soul," Best Poems Encyclopedia, accessed July 17, 2023, https://www.best-poem.net/poem/dark-night-by-john-cross.html.

[34] "Theodore Roosevelt Quotes," Goodreads, accessed July 25, 2023, https://www.goodreads.com/quotes/233139-courage-is-not-having-the-strength-to-go-on-it.

[35] Bragg and Bragg, *The Miracle of Fasting*, 105.

[36] Bragg and Bragg, 98.

[37] Leder, *More Beautiful Than Before*, 156.

[38] "Booker T. Washington Quotes," Goodreads, accessed July 25, 2023, https://www.goodreads.com/quotes/3189-i-have-learned-that-success-is-to-be-measure.

[39] Wolfe, *Healthy to 100*, 90.

[40] Morse, *The Detox Miracle Sourcebook*, 94–95.

[41] "George S. Patton Quotes," BrainyQuote, accessed July 24, 2023, https://www.brainyquote.com/quotes/george_s_patton_122094.

[42] Brene Brown, qtd on Carrots 'n' Cake, March 30, 2021, https://carrotsncake.com/one-day/.

[43] "Resilience Quotes," Goodreads, from *Resilience: Hard-Won Wisdom for Living a Better Life* by Eric Greitens (Irvine, CA: Harvest House, 2016), accessed July 29, 2023, https://www.goodreads.com/work/quotes/42099811-resilience-hard-won-wisdom-for-living-a-better-life.

[44] "John Salzgeber Quotes," Goodreads, accessed July 29, 2023, https://www.goodreads.com/quotes/10009048-no-tree-becomes-deep-rooted-and-sturdy-unless-strong-winds-blow.

[45] Angie Collins-Burke, RN, and Suzanne Cronkwright, "The Challenges of Living with an Invisible Illness: How to Cope with Questions, Judgment, Fatigue, and Guilt," Psychology Today, April 17, 2021, https://www.psychologytoday.com/us/blog/stroke-awareness/202104/the-challenges-living-invisible-illness.

[46] "Bobby Unser Quotes," BrainyQuote, accessed July 25, 2023, https://www.brainyquote.com/quotes/bobby_unser_126431.

ABOUT THE AUTHOR

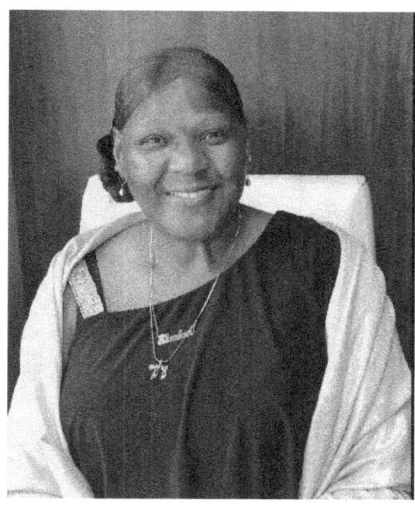

Dawn G. Green is a recovering Library Media Specialist with over 23 years' experience working with students and adults. She is an avid reader and has become an aficionado health expert, clocking over 20,000 research and study hours of the human body in her quest for answers to her health challenges.

As an inspiring author, Dawn is on a mission to share her extraordinary healing journey with the world and promote the importance of advocating for doctors to listen to their patients. This memoir is a powerful testament to her indomitable spirit. Join her on this profound journey of resilience, redemption, and self-discovery.

When not doing extensive research, Dawn Green enjoys spending time with her family and friends. She also loves traveling, going to the theatre and museums, playing board games, studying Hebrew, and doing arts and crafts.

Dawn resides in Virginia with her husband of 32 years, her college-aged daughter, and their dog, Spark.

www.ingramcontent.com/pod-product-compliance
Lightning Source LLC
Chambersburg PA
CBHW060527130626
46553CB00002B/673